TV, FOOD MARKETING AND CHILDHOOD OBESITY

TV, FOOD MARKETING AND CHILDHOOD OBESITY

JASON Y. CARTERE
EDITOR

Nova Science Publishers, Inc.
New York

LIBRARY OF CONGRESS CATALOGING-IN-PUBLICATION DATA

TV, food marketing and childhood obesity / editor, Jason Y. Cartere.
    p. cm.
  Includes index.
  ISBN 978-1-60692-196-8 (softcover)
  1. Obesity in children. 2. Food industry and trade. 3. Television advertising. I. Cartere, Jason Y.
  RJ399.C6T8 2009
  618.92'398--dc22
                            2008052170
  ISBN: 978-1-60692-196-8

Published by Nova Science Publishers, Inc. ✝ New York

CONTENTS

PREFACE

Obesity has become a major health concern in the U.S. and other countries as overweight and obesity rates have increased markedly since the early 1980s. The rise in children's obesity is a particular concern, because overweight children are more likely to become overweight adults, and because obese children are likely to suffer from associated medical problems earlier in life. Food marketing is among the postulated contributors to the rise in obesity rates. Food marketing to children has come under particular scrutiny because children may be more susceptible to marketing and because early eating habits may persist. Some researchers report that children's exposure to television advertising has been increasing along with the rise in children's obesity rates. This book presents a comprehensive analysis of the exposure of children to television advertising.

Chapter 1 - Childhood obesity rates in the United States have increased dramatically over the past two decades, posing serious health risks for children. In July 2005, the Federal Trade Commission ("FTC") and the Department of Health and Human Services ("HHS") (collectively "the agencies") held a public workshop to consider what the private sector can and should do to help lower childhood obesity rates. The workshop reviewed current food marketing practices and examined the actions that the food industry and media are taking to create and market healthier foods to children and to encourage positive changes in children's diets and health. It also examined current self-regulatory efforts governing food marketing to children. Workshop participants expressed both praise and criticism of existing industry practices and self-regulatory efforts. Some also offered suggestions for ways that industry can build on current efforts and take new steps to tackle the childhood obesity problem.

Chapter 2 - Obesity has become a major health concern in the U.S. and other countries as overweight and obesity rates have increased markedly since the early

1980s. The rise in children's obesity is a particular concern, because overweight children are more likely to become overweight adults, and because obese children are likely to suffer from associated medical problems earlier in life.

Food marketing is among the postulated contributors to the rise in obesity rates. Food marketing to children has come under particular scrutiny because children may be more susceptible to marketing and because early eating habits may persist. Some researchers report that children's exposure to television advertising has been increasing along with the rise in children's obesity rates.

This chapter presents a comprehensive analysis of the exposure of children, ages 2–11, to television advertising based on copyrighted Nielsen Monitor-Plus/Nielsen Media Research audience data from the 2004 television programming season. The detailed data covers the individual advertisements shown during four weeks of national and local ad-supported programming and includes paid commercials, public service announcements, and promotions for television programming. These data are projected to annual estimates.

Thirty years ago similar assessments of children's television advertising were done for the Federal Trade Commission's 1978 Children's Advertising Rulemaking. Since these research reports were done before the rise in children's obesity, they provide a baseline to measure changes in children's exposure to television advertising.

Since the late 1970s, other marketing has likely changed and new forms of marketing have emerged, including Internet-based advertising techniques. This chapter does not cover these marketing activities, but the FTC is in the process of conducting another study to attempt to gauge the extent of all forms of marketing to children.[1]

This chapter can also be used to measure future changes in children's exposure to television advertising as industry, parents, and children react to these health concerns.

In: TV, Food Marketing and Childhood Obesity   ISBN 978-1-60692-196-8
Editor: Jason Y. Cartere, pp.1-94   © 2009 Nova Science Publishers, Inc.

Chapter 1

PERSPECTIVES ON MARKETING, SELF-REGULATION, AND CHILDHOOD OBESITY[*]

Deborah Platt Majoras, Pamela Jones Harbour,
Jon Leibowitz, William E. Kovacic, J. Thomas Rosch and
Michael O. Leavitt

ABSTRACT

Childhood obesity rates in the United States have increased dramatically over the past two decades, posing serious health risks for children. In July 2005, the Federal Trade Commission ("FTC") and the Department of Health and Human Services ("HHS") (collectively "the agencies") held a public workshop to consider what the private sector can and should do to help lower childhood obesity rates. The workshop reviewed current food marketing practices and examined the actions that the food industry and media are taking to create and market healthier foods to children and to encourage positive changes in children's diets and health. It also examined current self-regulatory efforts governing food marketing to children. Workshop participants expressed both praise and criticism of existing industry practices and self-regulatory efforts. Some also offered suggestions for ways that

---

[*] A Report on a Joint Workshop of the Federal Trade Commission & the Department of Health & Human Services.

industry can build on current efforts and take new steps to tackle the childhood obesity problem.

Current Food Marketing to Children

The workshop found that food companies market their products to children using a wide variety of approaches. Traditional advertising in television and print media represents only one method of marketing food to children. Food marketers also reach children through packaging, labeling, promotional efforts like premiums and contests, product placement in movies and video games, branded advergaming, licensing of popular children's characters, and other tie-ins with children's movies and television programs. The use of these marketing techniques appears to be increasing.

Some workshop participants raised the concern that all of these techniques for marketing food to children are contributing to increasing rates of childhood obesity. There was wide agreement at the workshop that many factors contribute to childhood obesity. The purpose of the workshop was not to determine whether or to what extent food marketing, or any other single factor, has contributed to the dramatic rise in childhood obesity rates. Workshop participants generally agreed that, regardless of the causes of childhood obesity, responsible food marketers can use a wide range of methods to play a positive role in improving children's diets. There also was recognition that consumers expect industry to help families improve their diets and lifestyles. Workshop participants acknowledged that consumers not only want more choices and more nutrition information, they also want industry to market responsibly. The workshop explored ways to encourage forms of marketing that make a positive impact on children's health.

Some Recent Changes in Food Marketing Practices

Individual food companies at the workshop outlined changes in their marketing practices made to respond to rising childhood obesity rates. Many of them have introduced innovative products that are lower in calories and more nutritious. Some food companies have also modified their packaging to encourage portion control and make nutritious foods more convenient for parents and more appealing to children. Several of the companies participating in the workshop indicated that they are using labeling icons and seals to help consumers identify more nutritious, lower-calorie foods. Many food companies also reported that they are emphasizing nutrition and healthy lifestyle messages in advertising, using marketing techniques popular with children, such as character licensing, to promote good nutrition, and engaging in nutrition and fitness outreach programs in local communities and schools. Finally, a few food companies are limiting their child-directed advertising to products meeting specific nutrition and calorie standards.

These responses to childhood obesity, however, are only in their nascence. Consumer advocates and public health groups suggested that new offerings and reformulations do not go far enough and are still outweighed by poor nutritional offerings. They also expressed concern about whether multiple nutrition icons would be confusing to consumers and about whether food companies could be relied on to be persuasive or accurate with nutrition messages that might be at odds with some of the products they market. Participants were divided on the question of whether it is necessary or feasible to limit children's marketing to foods that meet certain nutritional standards.

After review of these examples of positive industry initiatives, and the suggestions and criticism of those outside of industry, the agencies recommend that food companies take the following actions:

- Intensify their efforts to create new products and reformulate existing products to make them lower in calories, more nutritious, more appealing to children, and more convenient to prepare and eat;
- Help consumers control portion sizes and calories through smaller portions, single- serving packages, and other packaging cues;
- Explore labeling initiatives, including icons and seals, to identify lower-calorie, nutritious foods clearly and in a manner that does not mislead consumers;
- Review and revise their marketing practices with the goal of improving the overall nutritional profile of the foods marketed to children, for example, by adopting minimum nutritional standards for the foods they market to children, or by otherwise shifting emphasis to lower-calorie, more nutritious products; and
- Generally explore ways to improve efforts to educate consumers about nutrition and fitness, with simple and effective messages.

Schools

Many food companies engage in a variety of marketing activities and sales in schools. Government studies have revealed that many of the foods sold competitively in schools, apart from the school meals programs, are high in calories and low in nutrition. To address concerns that have been raised about school marketing and sales, some food companies have decided to limit their marketing activities and restrict the foods they sell to more nutritious, lower-calorie products. The Institute of Medicine is currently developing nutritional standards for foods sold in schools as guidance for school districts and the food industry. The agencies recommend that all food companies review and revise their policies to improve the overall nutritional profile of the products they market and sell in schools.

Public Service Campaigns and Other Media Initiatives

Media and entertainment companies, like food companies, are changing their practices in response to rising childhood obesity rates by incorporating health and nutrition messages into programming and creating public education campaigns. The agencies recommend that, with broad participation from other stakeholders, the media and entertainment companies continue to develop and disseminate educational messages about nutrition and fitness that are simple, positive, and repeated consistently across various platforms and venues.

The entertainment industry has also begun to capitalize on the popularity of its television and movie characters to promote children's health. At the same time, critics point out that these characters are often used to sell foods that are high in calories and low in nutrition. The agencies recommend that companies review and revise their licensing of children's television and movie characters to foster promotion of more nutritious, lower-calorie foods.

Marketing to Racial/Ethnic Communities

The workshop also examined marketing of foods to certain racial and ethnic populations with a higher prevalence of childhood obesity. Addressing obesity in the Hispanic and African American communities is critical to decreasing the overall incidence of childhood obesity. Most childhood obesity initiatives to date have been directed at the general population. The agencies recommend that food companies make a concerted effort to include, as part of their marketing of more nutritious, lower-calorie foods, promotions that are tailored to specific racial and ethnic minority populations in which childhood obesity is more prevalent. The agencies also recommend that food companies, the media, and entertainment companies tailor their public education programs and other outreach efforts to promote better nutrition and fitness to these racial and ethnic minority populations.

Industry-Wide Self-Regulation

In addition to the actions of individual companies, the workshop examined self-regulatory efforts to ensure responsible food marketing to children. Participants focused on the Children's Advertising Review Unit ("CARU") of the Council of Better Business Bureaus, Inc. ("CBBB") and its guides requiring that advertising to children be truthful, accurate, and developmentally appropriate. Several suggestions were made at the workshop for expanding and enhancing the role of CARU to make it more effective in addressing food marketing to children, including a formal proposal by the food industry. These suggestions included updating and expanding the scope of CARU's authority to more explicitly cover newer forms of marketing, like the Internet and interactive games; ensuring that CARU has adequate resources and staff; and making the self-regulatory process more accessible to the public. Some also called for CARU to establish nutritional standards for foods marketed to children.

Although the CARU Guides are a good foundation for industry self-regulation, the agencies believe the guides should be expanded and their enforcement enhanced. The National Advertising Review Council ("NARC"), which sets policy and direction for CARU, has already taken some initial steps to address suggestions made at the workshop. As part of this review process, NARC and the CBBB recently formed a self-regulatory working group and have announced that the group intends to meet with various stakeholders as it develops proposals to modify the CARU Guides and to seek public input on any recommendations it makes. The agencies recommend that, as part of this effort, the CBBB/CARU working group take the following actions, as soon as practicable:

- Expand the CARU advisory board to include additional individuals with expertise in the
- various fields related to childhood obesity, such as nutrition, children's health, and developmental psychology;

- Allow parents and others to file complaints with CARU and make decisions more readily available to the public online; and
- Evaluate and determine whether CARU's staff and resources are sufficient to monitor and enforce adequately the CARU guides, in light of any changes made in response to the recommendations set forth in this chapter.

The agencies also recommend that, in addition to these actions, the CBBB/CARU working group also needs to consider a wide range of additional options as to how the CARU Guides could be modified to assist in combating childhood obesity. Among other things, the agencies recommend that the industry address the following issues:

- The scope of marketing activities covered by self-regulation, other than traditional advertising;
- The feasibility of minimum nutritional standards for foods marketed to children or other measures to improve the overall nutritional profile of foods marketed to children;
- The feasibility of an independent third-party seal or logo program identifying more nutritious, lower-calorie foods;
- Whether the use of product placement of foods is appropriate in certain media; and
- What additional sanctions or other measures should be incorporated into the CARU Guides to deter violations, especially repeated violations.

The agencies believe that improvements in each of these areas would be beneficial and that the CBBB/CARU working group should establish a process that is as open and transparent as possible, with broad participation by stakeholders to resolve these issues.

Report on Food Marketing

The workshop record indicates that food companies market their products to children through a variety of means, including television, radio, print and Internet advertising, packaging, promotional events, in-store marketing, and product placement. Preliminary research by the FTC staff suggests that children today are exposed to fewer food advertisements on television than in the past. There is less information, however, about the extent of other forms of marketing. A recently completed evidentiary review and analysis of food marketing and children's diets and health by the Institute of Medicine's Committee on Food Marketing and the Diets of Children and Youth (the "IOM Committee") noted significant gaps in the research. In particular, the IOM Committee's report notes that much of the relevant marketing research and data are proprietary and were not available to Committee members. It also noted that peer- reviewed literature on the role of food marketing in the diets of children is largely limited to television advertising and has not explored other marketing venues and techniques.

The FTC was recently directed by Congress to conduct a comprehensive food marketing study that will look at the full range of food marketing activities and expenditures directed at children and adolescents, drawing on both publicly available information and, as necessary, proprietary information from food companies. When completed, this study should provide a better understanding of the full extent and variety of techniques used to reach children. As described above, however, the agencies believe that there are many positive steps that individual food companies, and the private sector as a whole, can take now. The seriousness of the childhood obesity problem warrants such immediate action.

Conclusion

The agencies believe that the discussions of food marketing and childhood obesity at the workshop have created momentum to enhance self-regulation and industry practices that promote better children's diets. The agencies will monitor future developments in food marketing to children and childhood obesity and will closely evaluate the changes that the CBBB/CARU working group makes to the self-regulatory process, including assessing whether these changes satisfactorily address the specific recommendations in this chapter. After allowing time for changes to be implemented, one or both of the agencies will issue a follow-up report assessing the extent to which positive, concrete measures have been implemented and identifying what, if any, additional steps may be warranted to ensure adequate progress is being made to address childhood obesity.

ACRONYMS

AAAA	American Association of Advertising Agencies
AAF	American Advertising Federation
ABA	American Beverage Association
ACFN	American Council for Fitness and Nutrition
ADA	American Dietetic Association
ANA	Association of National Advertisers
CARU	Children's Advertising Review Unit
CBB	Council of Better Business Bureaus
CCFC	Campaign for a Commercial Free Childhood
CDC	Centers for Disease Control and Prevention
CIFC	Center for Informed Food Choices
CSPI	Center for Science in the Public Interest
CSS/GES	Collier Shannon Scott/Georgetown Economic Services
FCC	Federal Communications Commission
FDA	Food and Drug Administration
FNS	USDA Food and Nutrition Service
FTC	Federal Trade Commission
HHS	Department of Health and Human Services
GAO	Government Accountability Office (previously General Accounting Office)
GMA	Grocery Manufacturers of America
ICC	International Chamber of Commerce
IOM	Institute of Medicine of the National Academy of Sciences
NAD	National Advertising Division of the Council of Better Business Bureaus
NARB	National Advertising Review Board
NARC	National Advertising Review Council
NIH	National Institutes of Health
PBH	Produce for Better Health Foundation
PHAI	The Public Health Advocacy Institute
PMA	Promotion Marketing Association
USDA	United States Department of Agriculture

FEDERAL TRADE COMMISSION AND DEPARTMENT OF HEALTH AND HUMAN SERVICES WORKSHOP REPORT.[1]

I. INTRODUCTION

Obesity[2] among children in the United States is increasing rapidly. Since 1980, obesity rates have tripled among adolescents (ages 13 to 17) and doubled among younger children, with recent data indicating that 16% of children ages 6 to 19 years are obese.[3] In addition, not only have obesity rates increased, but the heaviest children are markedly heavier than they have been in the past.[4] Childhood obesity rates also are much higher in certain minority populations, particularly in the African-American and Hispanic communities, than in the general population.[5]

Childhood obesity is a significant public health problem,[6] because it raises serious and long-term disease risks. About 60% of obese children ages 5 to 10 years have at least one additional cardiovascular risk factor, such as elevated cholesterol, elevated insulin, elevated glucose, or elevated blood pressure. Twenty-five percent of obese children have two or more of these risk factors.[7] The health consequences of childhood obesity are compounded because it often persists into adulthood.[8] Obesity in adults is associated with diseases such as atherosclerosis, hypertension, cardiovascular disease, stroke, type II diabetes, hyperlipidemia, and arthritis. In addition to decreasing quality of life, obesity also has economic consequences. Recent estimates suggest that the total cost to Americans of obesity and associated health conditions was $117 billion in 2000.[9]

The federal government has undertaken many initiatives to reverse rising obesity rates, particularly among children. Because parents exercise control over many of the food choices of their children, especially younger children, providing nutrition and other information about foods to parents is well-recognized as a critical means of helping them make better decisions.[10] Last year, HHS, in combination with the United States Department of Agriculture ("USDA"), issued the 2005 Dietary Guidelines for Americans, which emphasize balancing calorie consumption with physical activity.[11] As part of the Food Guidance System, USDA has also created educational materials for children. "My Pyramid for Kids" includes an interactive computer game, tips for families, and classroom materials designed to help children ages 6 to 11 make healthy eating and physical activity choices.[12] Also in 2005, the National Institutes of Health ("NIH") launched "We Can," a national nutrition and fitness education program focusing on children ages 8 to 13. The program provides parents with information that encourages healthy eating and a more active lifestyle.[13]

Some of these initiatives are undertaken in partnership with non-governmental organizations. For example, the *"VERB. It's What You Do"* campaign is a national, multi cultural social marketing campaign coordinated by the Centers for Disease Control and Prevention ("CDC"). The campaign combines paid advertising, marketing strategies, and a variety of partnership efforts to reach young people ages 9 to 13.[14] Also, in October 2004, HHS signed a Memorandum of Understanding ("MOU") with the Girl Scouts of America to educate girls about obesity, and under the MOU the Food and Drug Administration ("FDA") is working with the Girl Scouts on healthy living initiatives.[15]

Several other government initiatives target obesity in the general population with nutrition and health messages for the whole family. In 2003, for instance, HHS launched the "Steps to a HealthierUS" initiative in support of President Bush's HealthierUS goal of helping all Americans live longer, better, and healthier lives. This wide-ranging initiative identifies and encourages modest behavior changes, like taking the stairs instead of the elevator, which can yield significant results over time.[16] In addition, the FDA has an initiative to make food labeling a more effective tool for managing calories. The FDA is considering modifying the food labeling regulations to give more prominence to calories and to revise its approach to serving size information. The FDA is encouraging marketers to modify their labels voluntarily while these proposed regulatory changes are under consideration.[17] In addition, the FDA is promoting better access to calorie and nutrition information in restaurants. The agency has funded a Keystone National Dialogue[18] to seek consensus-based solutions to specific aspects of the obesity problem related to away-from-home foods, which account for about 46% of the total food budget of Americans and a significant portion of total calories consumed.[19] In connection with this effort, the FDA has been encouraging restaurants to voluntarily provide consumers with caloric information at point of purchase, and encouraging consumers to ask for this information.[20]

The FTC's efforts to combat obesity include aggressive law enforcement actions against those who make false or misleading claims in advertising for weight loss products. Over the past decade, the Commission has brought over 100 cases targeting deceptive weight loss claims made for a variety of products and programs and has been successful in obtaining strong remedies in these cases.[21] The FTC recently has supplemented its traditional law enforcement activity by enlisting the assistance of the media to screen and reject weight loss ads with clearly deceptive claims.[22] These media screening efforts appear to be reducing the prevalence of the most deceptive claims for weight loss products.[23]

Despite these and other government initiatives, childhood obesity remains a serious public health problem. Some have contended that food marketing (including food advertising) is responsible for the recent increases in childhood obesity, and that, therefore, the government should ban or restrict food marketing to children. The FTC's experience in the 1970's with proposals to regulate food advertising on television directed to or seen by children[24] suggests that it would be difficult for the government to develop advertising restrictions that are practical and effective. In addition, tailoring such restrictions to conform to First Amendment constraints could present significant challenges.[25]

Instead, the FTC and HHS have decided to focus on identifying ways the government can encourage industry to harness its marketing power to generate solutions to childhood obesity.[26] On July 14 and 15, 2005, the agencies convened a public workshop to discuss steps that industry is taking and should take to decrease childhood obesity.[27]

The goal of the workshop was to "identify some concrete steps that industry, government, and public policy groups can take together to make progress against childhood obesity."[28] The workshop provided the food, beverage, and restaurant industries[29] and the media and entertainment industries with an opportunity to describe the changes they have made in their marketing and other practices to improve children's health,[30] and other interested parties with a chance to discuss the merits of these changes.[31] It prompted a critical examination of current self-regulatory standards for the marketing of foods to children.[32] This chapter summarizes the issues discussed at the workshop, draws conclusions, and makes recommendations regarding changes in company practices and industry self-regulation that may advance the common goal of decreasing childhood obesity.[33] It generally is based on the record of the workshop, including the presentations and discussions of panelists and other presenters and written comments submitted to the agencies, although it also notes some important developments that have occurred since the workshop. (A copy of the workshop agenda, including a list of panelists and presenters is attached as Appendix A.) In preparing this chapter the staff of the FTC and HHS did not attempt to look beyond the record of the workshop or to conduct their own research or literature review on food marketing and childhood obesity.[34]

II. OVERVIEW OF FOOD MARKETING TO CHILDREN

Food companies market their products to children using a wide variety of approaches. Traditional advertising in television and print media represents only part of marketing food to children.[35] Food marketers also reach children through packaging, labeling, promotional efforts like premiums and contests, product placement in movies and video games, branded advergaming, licensing of popular children's characters, and other tie-ins with children's movies and television programs.[36] With the increasing use of tie-ins and character licensing by the food industry, and the resulting association between these characters and specific food brands, some have argued that children's movies and programs may have become, themselves, an indirect form of marketing food to children.[37]

Children and adolescents are an important market segment. They not only have significant spending power of their own,[38] but they also influence the purchases of their parents and are the adult consumers of the future. The Institute of Medicine of the National Academy of Sciences ("IOM") has cited to research from the 1990s estimating children's purchasing influence rises with age, from $15 billion per year for children ages 3 to 5 years, to $90 billion per year for teens ages 15 to 17.[39] Much of that purchasing influence relates to food. According to one estimate, annual sales of foods to children exceeded $27 billion in 2002.[40]

It has been estimated that, because of children's impact on purchasing behavior, the food industry spent $10 to $12 billion in 2002 to reach them.[41] A substantial proportion of this amount is spent on a variety of promotions, contests, sweepstakes, and similar activities.[42] Food companies engage in promotional spending to draw the attention of their customers, including children, to specific products in the grocery store. For instance, food companies often pay a premium to grocery stores or other retailers to have their products placed on lower shelves, end- caps, or at check-out – all locations accessible to children.[43] Food companies also include prizes with their foods to make them more appealing to children. McDonald's, for example, has included Hot Wheels toy cars, Barbie dolls, and toys tied to Disney movies in its Happy Meals.[44] The Kellogg Company also has run an online promotion called "Magic by the Million" in which consumers enter the UPC symbol from a package of Keebler cookies or crackers into an on-line form to get the chance to win a Keebler cookie clip or a coupon for Keebler cookies.[45]

Another form of food promotion involves linking foods to popular children's characters or associating food brands with children's books, toys, and clothing. For example, Mattel sells a Barbie doll that wears a Jell-O Tee-shirt, as well as another doll dressed in a McDonald's restaurant uniform;[46] Scholastic publishes The M&M Counting book;[47] and Coke-branded toys include checker sets and cars purportedly aimed at children as young as 4.[48]

Tie-ins to popular children's movie and television characters may allow marketers to leverage children's frequent exposure to and familiarity with those characters. Kraft, for example, markets its Macaroni & Cheese in the shape of popular kids' characters, such as Super Mario Brothers, Flintstones, Bugs Bunny and Friends, Rugrats, Pokémon, Blues' Clues, Scooby Doo! and SpongeBob SquarePants.[49] Use of such characters may allow food companies to spend substantially less on advertising in television and other media.[50] For example, media spending for General Mills' Betty Crocker Fruit Snacks dropped from $6.6 million in 1998 to $26,000 in 1999, after General Mills, as part of a deal with Walt Disney, Co., introduced Winnie-the-Pooh, Mickey Mouse, and Disney Princess-based fruit snacks.[51]

Some workshop participants also emphasized the increased use of paid product placement in family programming on television,[52] as well as in movies, DVDs, and video games, as another technique used by food marketers. For example, in the *Spider-Man* movie, the protagonist used his web-spinning ability to retrieve a can of Dr. Pepper.

Food companies also spend significant amounts on packaging designed to appeal to children.[53] Food manufacturers use a variety of methods to make their packaging stand out to children, such as through the extensive use of color, the use of characters from popular movies and television shows, and the inclusion of toys.[54] Companies may also alter the size[55] and form of packaging to appeal to children. For instance, some ketchup bottles have been designed so that they are easier for children to squeeze.[56]

Food companies also spend substantial amounts on public relations to promote their corporate images and brand identities.[57] They donate money to schools in the form of corporate grants and gifts, distribute corporate-sponsored educational and teacher training materials, and conduct corporate-sponsored incentive programs.[58] Food companies also sponsor youth organizations, awards, scholarships, and healthy lifestyle programs.[59]

Finally, in addition to these marketing techniques, food companies spend significant amounts on traditional advertising to children.[60] Companies use a variety of advertising media to persuade parents and children to purchase their products, with television being the predominant choice. One advertising magazine has reported that, of the amount spent on advertising food to all consumers, 70% is spent on television advertising, 26% is spent on print advertising, 2% is spent on radio advertising, and slightly more than 1% is spent on online advertising.[61] Although these statistics are for food advertising to all consumers, not just children, they are consistent with the consensus of workshop participants that television advertising is the most visible form of traditional advertising that food companies use to reach children, as it has been for decades.

Workshop participants discussed whether the average number of television ads, including food ads, that children view has changed over the past three decades. A number of studies relating to this topic have been conducted with varying results.[62] At the workshop, Dr. Pauline Ippolito, Associate Director for the FTC's Bureau of Economics, presented preliminary results from a study on children's television ad exposure. She noted that, except for several studies in the 1970s, estimates of children's advertising exposure have been based on analyses of small subsets of programming. By contrast, the Bureau of Economics analyzed data on all programming monitored by Nielsen. The study analyzed Nielsen Monitor-Plus/Nielsen Media Research data on advertising viewed by children during four "sweeps" weeks in 2003-2004,[63] and compares it to similar analyses conducted in the late 1970s. The measures of ads viewed in 1977 are based on three prominent studies.[64]

The Bureau of Economics' preliminary analysis of results suggests that children's exposure to paid advertisements on television has declined from the late 1970s. Although children (ages 2-11) saw a total of approximately 22,000 ads per year in 1977 and an estimated 23,530 ads per year in 2004, the proportion of ads that were public service announcements and promotions for other television shows was considerably larger in 2004 than in 1977. Children saw an average of 17,507 paid ads in 2004, down from 20,000 in 1977.

The Bureau of Economics' preliminary analysis also suggests that children's exposure to television ads for foods has declined. On average, children saw nearly 5,000 nationally aired food ads on television in 2004. Children saw fewer food ads in 2004 than in 1977, but food ads continue to constitute a substantial percentage of the ads on children's shows[65] and family shows. According to the Bureau of Economics' analysis, the decline in food ads was offset primarily by increases in advertising for movies, DVDs, video games, computer games, and promotions for television programming.[66]

In addition to television advertising, online advertising of foods to children received significant attention at the workshop. Over the past decade, children have replaced some of their television viewing with time spent with other video media such as video games and the Internet.[67] Food companies have responded by creating websites with a variety of features that appeal to children.[68] Specifically, these websites may include interactive games that feature particular food products (sometimes referred to as "advergames"), contests, music, viral marketing in the form of e-mailing cards to friends, television commercial clips, sweepstakes, recipes, and downloadable wallpaper and screen savers.[69] Online advertising likely accounts for a minimal proportion of the total amount spent advertising food to children – reportedly slightly more than 1% of total advertising dollars spent on food in 2004.[70] On the other hand, some workshop participants cautioned that such expenditure data may understate the effect of online marketing to children, because children can become immersed in these websites and the activities available on them.[71]

Some have raised the concern that all of these techniques for marketing food to children are contributing to increasing rates of childhood obesity. There was wide agreement at the workshop that many factors other than marketing contribute to childhood obesity.[72] The purpose of the workshop was not to determine whether or to what extent food marketing, or any other single factor, has contributed to the recent and dramatic rise in childhood obesity rates.

Workshop participants generally agreed that, regardless of the causes of childhood obesity, responsible food marketers can use a wide range of methods to play a positive role in reversing obesity trends.[73] There also was recognition that consumers expect industry to help families improve their diets and lifestyles. Workshop participants acknowledged that consumers not only want more choices and more nutrition information, they also want industry to market responsibly. The workshop explored ways to encourage forms of marketing that make a positive impact on children's health.[74]

III. FOOD INDUSTRY INITIATIVES TO IMPROVE CHILDREN'S DIETS AND HEALTH

The record of the workshop shows that food companies are responding to rising childhood obesity rates with a variety of product changes and marketing initiatives. Product innovations include new product introductions, product reformulation, and changes in serving sizes and packaging. On the marketing side, companies report using labeling, advertising, and other marketing techniques to promote these healthier or lower-calorie products and to provide nutrition and health information to consumers. Some companies state that they also are limiting where and what they market to children. For instance, a number of companies have adopted policies limiting marketing in schools. Others are shifting much of their children's advertising to products meeting certain nutritional standards. Several companies are also engaging in outreach and educational programs in local communities and in schools.

Some members of the food industry emphasized that companies need to preserve some latitude as they experiment with how to make healthier products that will be successful in the marketplace. Market success, they contend, will spur competition to create more nutritious or lower-calorie products. They also stressed that companies need to experiment with different ways to market nutrition through labeling, advertising, and other marketing techniques. By trying different approaches, companies will learn what resonates best with parents and children.

It is not clear what impact these efforts to change products and marketing will have on childhood obesity. Some participants documented the success of new product lines that in turn are spurring additional product development. There was also some evidence indicating positive changes in consumer awareness and eating habits due to industry efforts, but this evidence was limited.

Other participants, however, expressed concern about the continuing imbalance between the extensive marketing and sale of foods of poor nutritional quality to children and the more limited efforts by industry and others to promote children's health. They argued further that, in some instances, reformulated products are not necessarily healthier, because they remain high in sugar or have other unhealthy attributes. These participants also expressed concern about the usefulness of nutrition seal programs used to promote healthier and lower-calorie products, questioned the effectiveness of company policies that purport to limit advertising to children, and contended that company-sponsored outreach programs on health and nutrition are potentially misleading and may be just another form of marketing to children.

A. Products and Packaging

Consumers indicate that they want nutritious and low-calorie options, and the marketplace appears to be responding to that demand.[75] According to a survey by the Grocery Manufacturers of America ("GMA") of industry's self-reported health and wellness initiatives, new and recently reformulated offerings represent about 30% of the average supermarket offerings.[76] Product and packaging innovation includes new products that are lower in calories or more nutritious; products that have been reformulated to reduce or eliminate sugars or unhealthy fats; portions that are smaller; and packaging that offers smaller serving sizes.[77] All can provide direct benefits toward reducing obesity.

The challenge for food companies is to create lower-calorie, more nutritious products that will be successful with consumers. Although consumers say they want healthy options, according to industry participants, consumers do not always choose these options when they are made available. The restaurant industry reports, for example, that larger portions in restaurants connote value and consumers sometimes reject reduced portion sizes as poor value.[78] To be a market success, lower-calorie, more nutritious offerings also need to taste good and offer convenience.[79] In the case of children's products, industry participants stated that it is equally important that their products be seen as fun or "cool."[80] As one participant noted, if a product is nutritious, but not good tasting and fun, it stays in the cupboard and does not improve children's diets.[81]

1. New Products and Reformulations

Several companies reported on their efforts to create new products that are lower in calories or more nutritious. Coca-Cola, for example, indicated that it has introduced 15 new low- calorie or calorie-free beverages in the past year and that its fastest growing portfolio of brands within the company is bottled water.[82] Similarly, Pepsi indicated that 50% of its new product development will be products that meet the company's "Smart Spot" nutritional standards, and Kraft reported that much of its new product growth is in the category of products meeting its "Sensible Solutions" nutrition standards.[83] Many of the industry's new product offerings are specifically targeted to children. McDonald's now offers apple slices and low-fat milk as a substitute for french fries and soft drinks in its Happy Meals.[84] Kellogg's has introduced new whole grain children's cereals, such as Kashi Mighty Bites.[85]

Companies are also reformulating existing products to make them lower in calories and more nutritious. The most common reformulations involve reducing or eliminating saturated fat and trans fat, decreasing calories, increasing whole grain content, or reducing sugar content.[86] McDonald's, for instance, pointed to its introduction of its 100% white meat chicken nuggets.[87] Kellogg's noted that it has reformulated its Frosted Flakes and Fruit Loops cereals to reduce sugar content, introduced a low-fat version of its Nutri-Grain waffles, offered sugar-free varieties of its cookies, and removed trans fat from its Rice Krispies Treats.[88] With their new product development, Kraft and Pepsi cited efforts to create reformulated products that conform to internal nutritional standards so that more of their overall portfolios will qualify for their healthier Sensible Solution and Smart Spot marketing initiatives, respectively.[89] General Mills also has implemented an initiative to convert all of its cereal products to whole grain.[90]

To make it more likely that these new products will succeed, companies plan to actively advertise and promote them with campaigns that focus on good nutrition. Kraft, for example, has indicated that its advertising to children of its Sensible Solution products will highlight nutrition whenever practical.[91] Pepsi is planning an educational campaign founded on its Smart Spot program to teach consumers simple tips for improving diet and health.[92]

Although participants recognized the value of offering healthier food options in the marketplace, some criticized industry efforts as inadequate or even deceptive in certain instances. They suggest that the changes do not go far enough and are still outweighed by the poor nutritional offerings on the market.[93] Some of the reformulated products, these participants

contend, are promoted heavily for their nutritional and health benefits and yet continue to be high in sugar or have other characteristics that these participants believe are unhealthy. For example, the Center for Informed Food Choices ("CIFC") contended that most of the General Mills whole grain cereals marketed to children, such as Reese's Puffs, Cookie Crisps, Cocoa Puffs, and Lucky Charms, continue to contain substantial amounts of sugar (sometimes as the primary ingredient) and little fiber. CIFC notes that whole grain Cocoa Puffs, for instance, contains 13 grams of sugar and only one gram of fiber.[94]

2. Packaging

Companies also are using packaging technologies in a variety of ways that may help improve consumer diets. Most companies reported making changes to both multi-serving and single-serving packaging to help consumers manage portions and calorie intake.[95] General Mills, for example, has introduced 100-calorie packs for some of its snack food products, like popcorn.[96] To help with portion control, General Mills also has redesigned packaging for products like frozen dinner rolls to allow consumers to bake only one or two at a time.[97] Pepsi, Coca-Cola, Kraft, Kellogg's, and many other companies also are moving to portion-controlled packages, including smaller, more child-appropriate sized beverages and snacks.[98]

Other packaging innovations include making nutritious foods more fun and appealing to children. For example, McDonald's repackaged its milk, changing from traditional wax cartons to brightly decorated and easily opened small plastic jugs, with the reported result that milk sales for the chain doubled.[99] General Mills claims to have been similarly successful with its Go-Gurt yogurt in a squeezable tube, to which it attributes a substantial increase in yogurt consumption by children ages 6 to 12.[100]

Finally, processing and packaging technologies are allowing companies to make fruit and vegetables more convenient for consumers.[101] General Mills, for example, is currently testing single-serving microwavable bowls of vegetables for both adults and children, and it reports a positive consumer response to these products.[102] Also, Dole Food Company has introduced its single-serving size Fruit Bowls containing bite-sized fruit pieces that do not require refrigeration.[103]

B. Labeling, Advertising, and other Promotions

In addition to product innovations, companies are using marketing to educate and motivate parents and children to eat better – through labeling, advertising, community-based outreach programs, and other means. Some companies now place icons or seals on their product packaging to identify foods that satisfy certain nutritional criteria. Companies also have adopted policies restricting their advertising to children; re-focused their advertising messages on nutrition and healthy lifestyles; and sponsored community outreach programs, particularly in schools, to promote healthy eating and exercise habits.

Regardless of the marketing method companies use to promote healthy eating, there was general agreement about the content of messages that resonate best with families. Many industry participants agreed that, for both parents and children, messages need to be simple and positive. Consumers, the companies suggested, want a clear signal to help them make better diet choices, without too much information or detail.[104] These participants further stated that parents in particular do not respond well to negative messages warning against unhealthy nutrients or messages that create guilt.[105] Likewise, they submitted that children do not respond well to lectures about nutrition. These participants said that messages that resonate best with children focus on having fun, being cool, having energy, and doing well in school and in sports.[106] Several participants emphasized the importance of consistent messaging throughout the marketplace and the need for constant, repeated exposure.[107] At the same time, some participants stated that diet and health messages may need to be tailored to specific ethnic groups and specific ages to have the greatest impact.[108]

1. Labeling

A significant trend in labeling is the development by some food companies of icons or seal programs. Marketers use these labeling tools as a quick and easy way to help consumers identify the most nutritious products in a brand line or to convey a nutritional benefit of a product.

In the past, seals typically have been issued by independent nonprofit and public health organizations, like the American Heart Association, to identify foods that meet certain health criteria. But many companies are now developing proprietary seal programs for use on their own products. Kraft and Pepsi also have both implemented seal programs for their healthier products. Kraft's "Sensible Solution" labeling program uses a flag on foods that meet specific "better-for you" criteria. The criteria for this program, independently developed by Kraft, include limits on, or reductions in, calories, fat, sugar, and sodium, the presence of beneficial nutrients like calcium or fiber, and the delivery of a functional benefit like heart health.[109] Pepsi has a similar seal program using a "Smart Spot" green dot on packaging to identify its "good-for-you" and "better-for-you" products. In deciding which products qualify for its Smart Spot seal, Pepsi uses nutritional criteria based on limits on, or reductions in, saturated fat, trans fat, cholesterol, sodium, and added sugar.[110] Kellogg's has also developed nutrition icons for its cereal packaging,[111] and General Mills has created a "Goodness Corner" icon system that appears on the front of its cereal boxes.[112] The icons identify particular nutritional benefits of the product, such as "good source of calcium." These benefits are founded, in part, on FDA criteria and guidelines for nutrients and in part on the companies' own criteria.

Food companies that use nutrition icons or seals on product packaging report that their programs have been well-received by consumers and have increased sales. Kraft indicated that sales of its Sensible Solution products are growing at a rate three to four times faster than its products that do not qualify for the flag. In addition, the program has created incentives within the company to develop products that qualify for the flag, with resulting improvement in the overall nutritional profile of Kraft's portfolio.[113] Similarly, Pepsi reported that its Smart Spot products were 39% of the product mix but represented 65% of the company's revenue growth in North America, and were growing at three times the rate of its other products.[114] The companies agree that these programs are popular with consumers, because, as company-sponsored focus groups and quantitative research suggest, consumers want simple messages without too much information or detail, and prefer clear, positive signals over negative information or warnings.[115]

Companies also reported that the icons seemed to resonate even more with consumers in lower socio-economic groups and in certain minority communities.[116] Thus, these labeling programs may be one way to reach specific populations that are at higher risk of obesity.

Some participants, however, criticized these seal programs. They expressed concern about the subjective nature of the nutritional criteria that companies apply and suggested that the seals were being used in some cases as a means of promoting sales of less nutritious foods to health-conscious consumers.[117] In addition, although there was general agreement that consumers find nutrition icons helpful, there was also recognition that having multiple health nutrition icons in the marketplace with different formats and meaning could potentially be confusing to consumers.[118] Such confusion could be confounded if terms were used in a manner inconsistent with those used for specific nutrient content claims approved for food labeling by the FDA.[119] Some participants agreed that it might be desirable at some point for companies to collaborate to create more consistency across seal programs, and some suggested that there was an immediate need to standardize these efforts.[120] At the same time, others pointed to the advantages of allowing experimentation by companies to learn what programs work best[121] for particular types of consumers or categories of products.[122] A one-size-fits-all system, for example, would not allow for programs that identified the relatively healthier offerings in a particular category of less nutritious foods like cookies.[123]

Nutrition seals and icons were the most common labeling initiatives reported by companies, but not the only examples of company efforts to educate consumers through enhanced labeling. Some companies reported that they were incorporating the 2005 USDA Food

Guidance System on their packaging,[124] and using games, trivia, and puzzles on cereal boxes and other packaging to teach children about nutrition.[125] Other approaches to enhanced labeling included providing clearer calorie information on the Nutrition Facts Panel on single-serving products[126] and indicating the number of servings per package on the front.[127] In addition, McDonald's recently announced its plans to place certain nutrition and calorie information on wrappers and boxes of some of its popular menu items.[128]

2. Advertising

Beyond labeling, many of the industry's efforts to change the way it markets foods to children have focused on television and other forms of traditional advertising, with less attention given to promotions and other marketing techniques. These changes in advertising fall within two general categories: 1) limits on advertising directed at children; and 2) advertising that incorporates educational messages about diet and healthy lifestyle.

a. Restrictions on Advertising to Children

Although most companies have not adopted voluntary restrictions on the ways they market or advertise food to children, some have. The Coca-Cola Company stated that it does not advertise its soft drinks to children under 12 and has not done so for 50 years.[129] Kraft reported that it has a longstanding policy not to advertise in TV, radio, or print media that primarily reach children under age 6. Further, the company is shifting the mix of products that it advertises in media primarily reaching children ages 6 to 11 to products it identifies as healthier under its nutrition standards.[130] Kraft indicated that, by the end of 2005, only those products meeting

Kraft's nutritional criteria for its Sensible Solutions program would be advertised in children's media.[131] Similarly, Pepsi indicated that it was committed to shifting its children's advertising to products meeting its Smart Spot criteria.[132]

Other companies are not applying any nutrition standards to limit the products they advertise in children's media. Moreover, some participants point out that even companies that have adopted voluntary limits on what they advertise to children are still reaching a significant number of children through other means. For example, even though the absolute number of children who view many prime time television shows may be large, voluntary limits on advertising to children do not address advertising on such shows, because children are not the primary viewing audience in terms of percentages.[133] Nor do these voluntary actions address promotional activities, like tie-ins with children's movies and television programs, branding of children's toys, Internet sites with company-branded games, or other marketing techniques that appeal to children.[134]

Participants and commenters were polarized on the question of whether nutritional standards for advertising directed to children should be adopted industry-wide. Many public health advocates and nutritionists stressed the need for such standards. The Produce for Better Health Foundation ("PBH"), a non-profit organization promoting more fruit and vegetable consumption, urged the FTC and HHS to develop national nutritional standards for foods that can be advertised and marketed to children.[135] The Center for Science in the Public Interest ("CSPI") suggested that the poor nutritional quality of products marketed to children is the central problem with current marketing practices and needs to be addressed systematically. CSPI has proposed nutritional guidelines for voluntary implementation by industry.[136] Others also urged consideration of such an approach.[137]

Some industry representatives rejected nutritional standards for advertising to children as "paternalistic," especially if imposed industry-wide, arguing that any food can be eaten in moderation as part of a well-balanced diet.[138] Even companies that successfully use nutritional criteria for their own marketing to children were skeptical about whether there is sufficiently broad support for a voluntary industry-wide approach to succeed at this time.[139] Section VI provides a more detailed discussion of proposals to create industry-wide nutritional standards for foods marketed to children, as part of a self-regulatory program.

b. Nutrition and Healthy Lifestyle Advertising

Some food companies also reported that they are shifting their advertising messages to focus more on nutrition and healthy lifestyles. For example, McDonald's asserted that a significant percentage of its advertising now focuses on balanced lifestyle messages, including an advertising campaign for children using Ronald McDonald and famous athletes, including Venus and Serena Williams, Tony Hawk, and others, to promote energy balance through diet and exercise.[140] Similarly, Kellogg's described a general policy of encouraging physical activity and exercise in its advertising to children whenever possible. It also discussed a number of educational marketing campaigns directed at children that include advertising and other marketing elements, such as the "Earn Your Stripes" campaign with Tony the Tiger and famous athletes promoting physical activity and good diet, and "Zumbando con Kellogg's," a campaign targeting the Hispanic community and using Latin music to promote dance, exercise, and a balanced diet.[141]

Although company-sponsored educational messages like these can help to reinforce the efforts of government and public health authorities to promote good nutrition, some participants questioned whether food companies can be relied on to give the most persuasive or accurate messages about diet. Those messages, they suggest, sometimes conflict with company efforts to market products that often are low in nutrition and high in calories.[142]

3. Other Marketing and Promotions

Food companies have successfully used in-store promotions, advergaming, licensing of children's characters, contests, and free samples to market their products to children. Food companies reported that they are now beginning to tap these resources more often for marketing good nutrition and exercise. PBH has partnered with National Institute of Health's National Cancer Institute and a number of restaurants, grocery stores, and other retailers to promote increased consumption of fruits and vegetables. One example is PBH's partnership with Wal-Mart for in-store promotional events using popular children's characters like Shrek, Charlie Brown, and Spider-Man. The events also include fruit and vegetable samples, free children's activity books, and other giveaways – techniques that have long been used by food marketers to make their products more appealing to children.[143] Such promotions at retail sites and restaurants, according to industry, show some promise in influencing children's diets.[144] PBH and its partners, for instance, have increased consumer awareness of the "5 A Day" program from 40% in 2003 to nearly 60% in 2005 and, as consumers have become more aware of the campaign, they have also begun to eat more fruit and vegetables.[145]

Food companies also stated that they are using the Internet to convey nutrition and fitness messages. Kidnetic.com, for example, is a children's fitness website created by the International Food Information Council, in partnership with health and fitness organizations, and financed by contributions from food and beverage companies. The site includes games, recipes, health tips, bulletin boards, and other activities on diet and health.[146] Other companies, like Kraft, report shifting the content of their websites and focusing web games more on health and wellness messages.[147]

4. Community Outreach and Education

In addition to making changes in how they market their products, several companies and industry groups said that they are sponsoring outreach programs in local communities and schools. Proponents of these community and school programs point out that the programs directly address obesity by actively engaging children and giving them tangible goals to exercise more and eat more healthfully.[148]

Often, these outreach efforts involve partnerships with local government or with health and nutrition advocates. Some of the programs reportedly have focused on specific minority populations, where childhood obesity is more prevalent. For example, the American Council for Fitness and Nutrition ("ACFN"), a non-profit organization whose members include food companies and health and nutrition advocates, has developed a number of community outreach programs, including two pilot programs in 2004 specifically targeted to Hispanic and African- American families.[149] In addition, several individual companies stated that they are also partnering with health and fitness groups to create and sponsor outreach programs.[150]

Some food marketers also explained that they have prepared educational materials for use in elementary and middle schools. For instance, Pepsi partnered with America On the Move to create the "Balance First" lesson plans and other materials to teach elementary and middle school children about balancing calorie intake with physical activity. The program reached three million elementary school students in 2004 and was scheduled to be distributed to 15,000 middle schools in 2005 in partnership with Discovery Education.[151] Similarly, Coca-Cola was set to launch its "Live-It" program, a nutrition and exercise program, in one-third of middle schools in the fall of 2005.[152] Both programs use non-branded materials in the schools.[153]

Some workshop participants expressed concern that the company-sponsored programs focus too much on exercise as a solution and not enough on avoiding high-calorie, low-nutrition foods, including those that are marketed by the food company sponsoring the programs.[154] Also, these participants charge, programs are often heavily branded and thus constitute another means of marketing to children. In addition, few of these programs include any means to evaluate outcomes, thus making it difficult to know how much impact they actually have.[155]

C. Marketing and Sale in Schools

Many companies engage in a variety of marketing activities and sales in schools. In 2004, the Government Accountability Office ("GAO") issued a report on commercial activities in schools documenting a range of direct advertising and indirect marketing. Examples include: signage and billboards in schools and on school buses and shelters; logos and brand names on school equipment such as marquees and scoreboards; logos, ads, and brand names on book covers, assignment books, and posters; ads in school publications; ads on Channel One and on Internet sites used within the school; free samples; and corporate-sponsored education materials, contests, incentives, and gifts.[156] In addition to these marketing activities, companies also sell foods and beverages in schools outside of the USDA-supervised school meal program. Sale of such foods in the school cafeteria alongside school meals, in vending machines, school stores, and snack bars is common at all grade levels.[157] Government studies and other reviews have noted that many of these foods are high in calories and low in nutrition. A 2001 report by USDA, for example, found foods sold in competition with school meal programs to be relatively low in nutrient density and relatively high in fat, added sugars, and calories.[158]

Some companies have begun to voluntarily address concerns about the marketing and sale of high-calorie, low-nutrition foods in schools. A few have cut back or eliminated marketing activities in the school setting, and some also have implemented nutritional standards for the foods they sell in schools. Kraft, for example, reports that it has eliminated all in-school advertising and promotion and has established nutritional guidelines for school vending machine sales, such as 10% or less of total calories from a combination of saturated and trans fat.[159] Coca- Cola has guidelines against the sale of carbonated beverages in elementary schools, but not in middle or high schools. In middle and high schools, the company points to a policy that more than half of offerings should be zero-calorie and non-carbonated beverages.[160] Pepsi recommends that all of the products sold by its distributors in elementary schools and a majority of products in other schools meet its Smart Spot nutritional criteria. The company also recommends to its distributors that elementary school offerings be limited to single-serve packs of less than 150 calories.[161] Finally, in August 2005, the American Beverage Association announced a school vending policy under which the beverage industry would voluntarily restrict beverage sales in elementary schools to only water and 100% juice. In middle schools, the policy would prevent the sale of full-calorie soft drinks or full-calorie juice drinks with less than 5% juice during the school day. In high schools, no more than 50% of vending selections would be soft drinks.[162]

Some participants view the industry's efforts to date as inadequate and question whether some of the initiatives represent real progress.[163] Participants point out that, despite company policies against marketing in schools, branding and other examples of marketing continue.[164] Many school vending machines, for example, have advertising panels on the front.[165] The mere selling of products in schools, one consumer advocate contends, is in itself a form of marketing. [166] Some participants also expressed concern about whether the voluntary nutritional standards that some companies have adopted for foods sold in school go far enough to eliminate foods that are low in nutrition and high in calories,[167] while others suggested that the restrictions become progressively too lenient at the middle school and high school level.[168] At the same time, at least one participant emphasized the importance of keeping in mind that school funding needs often are the underlying reason for commercial activities in schools.[169]

CDC has urged educators, families, school, and public health officials to work together to improve the school nutrition environment, characterizing the goal as "integral to any strategy to improve dietary behavior and reduce overweight among youths."[170] Local school districts, state legislatures, and the federal government all are responding with initiatives to create healthier school environments, including measures to require or encourage improvements in the nutritional quality of what is sold in schools. The 2004 GAO report indicated, for example, that 24 states had recently considered bills to restrict or ban the sale of beverages and foods of limited nutritional value in schools.[171] Congress has also taken action, establishing a new requirement that all school districts with a federally funded school meals program must develop and implement wellness policies that address nutrition and physical activity by the start of the 2006 2007 school year.[172] As part of these wellness policies, schools must set nutritional guidelines for all foods sold in schools outside of the school meals program. The requirement allows the local school districts to determine the specifics of any nutritional criteria.[173]

The most recent federal government initiative that directly relates to the industry's sale of foods in schools is an ongoing project by the IOM's Food and Nutrition Board. Congress directed CDC to conduct a study and make recommendations concerning appropriate nutrition standards for such foods, in part to assist schools as they develop their required 2006 wellness policies. The study, which began in August 2005, is being implemented by the IOM with a final report to be issued by October 2006.[174] The IOM Committee on Nutrition Standards for Foods in Schools includes members with expertise in nutrition, public health, and education. It is charged specifically with reviewing the data on the availability and nutritional profile of foods sold in schools and developing science-based nutritional standards for those foods. The standards recommended by the IOM committee are not a mandatory element of the wellness policy requirement for the 2006 school year, but could provide important guidance for local school districts as well as for the food industry.

IV. MEDIA AND ENTERTAINMENT INDUSTRY INITIATIVES TO IMPROVE CHILDREN'S DIETS AND HEALTH

Like the food industry, the media have an important role to play in educating children and parents about nutrition and physical activity and influencing behavior to help combat childhood obesity. Research indicates that television is the primary source of nutrition information for all ages[175] and estimates that 65% of all American children have a television in their room.[176] Members of the media are responding to rising obesity rates by developing public service announcement ("PSA") campaigns, donating money and air time for these campaigns, incorporating nutrition and fitness messages into programming, and licensing characters from children's programs to promote healthier food choices to children.

A. Public Service Campaigns and Program Content

Public service campaigns can educate children and parents about the importance of a nutritious diet and active lifestyle – two things that can help counter obesity. To be effective, workshop participants said, these campaigns need to have messages that are simple, consistent, and constantly reinforced.[177] One example of a public service campaign that was reportedly effective in communicating simple messages is the "Small Steps" campaign – a collaborative effort between the Ad Council and HHS. Launched in 2004, the campaign targets parents, as the role model for their families, suggesting a variety of small changes in behavior that can lead to better diet, more exercise, and improved health.[178] Over the course of the campaign, the Small Steps website has attracted more than one million visitors and gets an average of 80,000 visitors per month.[179]

Initial findings about the impact of the Small Steps campaign showed that, after ten months, public awareness of the actual PSAs and awareness of the Small Steps messages increased.[180] More people indicated that they were taking small steps to lead healthier lives. The campaign also resonated particularly with the Hispanic community, increasing awareness among Hispanics that small changes in eating habits and physical activities can have an impact on weight and health.[181] Although the findings suggest the media's potential to educate viewers and influence their choices, they did not indicate dramatic behavioral changes. Only slightly over a third of those surveyed were considering or actually making changes to their lifestyle.[182]

The Ad Council also spearheads The Coalition for Healthy Children initiative, which is a collaborative effort with several industry members.[183] The Ad Council created the coalition to develop consistent messaging for use in communications and to provide a mechanism for measuring the collective efforts of these sectors to change key attitudes and behaviors related to obesity.[184] The messages developed for this initiative are based on research on parents and children to determine what would be most motivating for behavioral change.[185] The Ad Council is monitoring the campaign's effect on attitudes and behavior through an on-going tracking study.[186]

Univision, a major network serving the Hispanic community, has also committed money and air time towards educating its viewers about health and wellness. Univision teamed up with HHS and public health groups such as the Kaiser Family Foundation to develop a public service campaign for the Hispanic community, *Salud Es Vida ... Enterate* (Lead a Healthy Life, Get the Facts). The campaign was launched in 2003, with PSAs airing across all of Univision's media, including two television networks, radio stations, and the Internet.[187]

Having consulted with experts in preschool health, nutrition, and pediatrics, Sesame Workshop launched "Healthy Habits for Life," an initiative based on in-house research regarding children's perceptions of the term "healthy."[188] The initiative includes English and Spanish PSAs featuring Sesame Street characters but goes beyond PSAs to encompass nutrition and fitness messages in television programming on the Public Broadcasting System, Internet materials, and DVDs. As one example of the effort, the Sesame Workshop has teamed with Sunkist to encourage children, with help from the Cookie Monster, to choose citrus fruit as a healthy snack.[189] The panelist from Sesame Workshop noted that because the emphasis of the campaign is on obesity prevention, as opposed to intervention, it targets a younger audience.[190]

The Ad Council said that commitment from media outlets to support public service campaigns is vital to their success. Because television advertising is very expensive, substantial financial support is necessary for PSAs developed by non-profit organizations to receive national air time. As one panelist pointed out, a commitment from media outlets of a significant amount of air time for PSAs helps ensure that messages can penetrate to audiences in a sustained way.[191] The Small Steps campaign, for example, received up-front commitments from national and local media for television air time, with more than $106 million donated for media coverage.[192] Nickelodeon commits 10% of its total media time annually, over $20 million, to nutritional literacy spots aimed at children and parents.[193] Nickelodeon also creates its own health and wellness spots to air on its channels, such as a new campaign that teaches children the importance of eating breakfast every morning, and the "Let's Just Play" campaign.[194] Let's Just Play also includes an initiative to prompt kids to be more active through partnerships with community-based organizations across the country that encourage physical activity.[195] Nickelodeon also recently expanded its Let's Just Play initiative to a nationwide partnership with the American Heart Association and the William J. Clinton Foundation. The partnership, The Alliance for a Healthier Generation, is launching a comprehensive media and public awareness campaign.[196]

Despite the reach of successful PSA campaigns, some participants expressed doubt that they can counter the large presence of food marketing to children.[197] The American Dietetic Association ("ADA") noted that its research indicates that educational messages about nutrition on television are insufficient to balance food marketing on television.[198] One panelist commented that, notwithstanding the positive effect public education campaigns have on young people, social campaigns face significant challenges, whether they are done through PSAs or commercial advertising.[199] For example, this panelist commented that promoting healthier foods and exercise to children tends to be a tougher sell than advertising for less nutritious foods, such as certain cereals, fast food, soft drinks, and snacks.[200] Another participant mentioned that, because the amount of food marketing is substantially greater than the amount of media time donated for PSAs, children see many more ads promoting foods high in calories and low in nutrition than ads promoting nutrition and fitness,[201] which makes it harder for PSAs to impact children's attitudes and behavior.[202] She further observed that, unlike the case with successful social marketing campaigns on other topics, children are exposed to "counter-advertising" that promotes less nutritious food choices and often makes such foods more appealing to children by touting their fun factor.[203] The panelist also suggested it is more challenging to persuade people to avoid behavior that is lawful, such as eating high-calorie foods, than it is to advocate against unlawful conduct, such as driving without a seatbelt or drunk driving.[204]

B. Licensing of Popular Characters

Several participants expressed concern about media's licensing of characters from popular movies and television shows to food companies to promote less nutritious foods. As noted earlier in this chapter, some workshop participants said that marketing and packaging featuring popular characters can successfully attract children to such foods and increase their appeal. Some research appears to confirm that popular characters can influence children's food choices. A participant from Sesame Workshop described research that paired different food items with Sesame Street characters to see how children reacted to the foods. The results suggest that when a familiar character, like Elmo, was paired with food items, it substantially increased the appeal of the food with which it was shown, whether broccoli or chocolate.[205] This suggests that popular characters can be used to promote more nutritious, lower-calorie foods to children.

Some media outlets have begun to license characters for the marketing of more nutritious, lower-calorie foods to children. Nickelodeon recently announced a new partnership that will pair some of its more popular characters with fruits and vegetables. Packaging for spinach and carrots will feature Nickelodeon's SpongeBob Squarepants, Dora the Explorer, and LazyTown characters.[206] Nickelodeon also plans to license characters from Blue's Clues, Dora the Explorer, and the Backyardigans to promote oranges.[207] In addition, Nickelodeon has partnered with the Produce for Better Health Foundation on its "5 A Day" campaign so that popular Nickelodeon characters can help spread the 5 A Day message to kids. Walt Disney has also indicated that it will begin to remove characters like Winnie the Pooh, Mickey Mouse, and Chicken Little from candy and other less nutritious foods and is partnering with a supermarket chain to place a Mickey Mouse seal on items like bananas, and certain store-brand juices and other foods.[208] Panelists agreed that using such characters to increase children's interest in healthier foods is a step in the right direction.[209]

V. FOOD AND BEVERAGE MARKETING TO MINORITY YOUTH

Research shows that obesity and the accompanying health problems disproportionately affect minority populations.[210] Obesity rates are increasing faster in certain groups than in the general population, particularly in the African-American and Hispanic communities. Given that minority youth are predicted to comprise almost half of all U.S. children by the year 2010,[211] decreasing childhood obesity in minority populations would result in a substantial decrease in overall childhood obesity levels. Consequently, participants often mentioned the specific impact on minorities of different types of marketing that target children, the steps that the food industry is taking to address childhood obesity, and the role of the media in educating children.

A. Advertising and Marketing

African-American and Hispanic children reportedly spend significantly more time watching television and viewing other media than non-Hispanic white children. One participant described a recent report of the Kaiser Family Foundation finding that African-American youth ages 8 to 18 spend 141/2 more hours per week and Hispanic youth spend six more hours per week watching television, DVDs, and movies than non-Hispanic white youth.[212] According to Dr. William Dietz of the CDC, these differences in media use among African-American and Hispanic youth mirror the disparities that are seen in obesity rates between these groups and the general population.[213] Dr. Dietz noted that this correlation does not necessarily imply a causal link between screen time and obesity, but suggests that it is a possible contributory factor.[214]

The type of television programming that minority children watch may also affect the nutritional profile of food products advertised to them. For example, it has been reported that television programs directed to African-American audiences contain a significantly higher percentage of ads for desserts, sweets, and soda compared to programs directed to general audiences.[215] This advertising, according to some participants, is also less likely to contain messages promoting health and wellness.[216] Similarly, other research indicates that, compared to magazines with a predominantly white readership, magazines targeted to minority audiences include more ads for less nutritious foods, such as snacks, desserts, soda, and fast food.[217]

One participant reported that minority children have been found to respond more favorably to ethnically targeted marketing strategies than to marketing that is designed for the general population.[218] The panelist stated that advertisers use racial and ethnic cues (such as minority models, ethnic symbols, linguistic styles, and music) to link cultural values, beliefs, and norms with brand names or with the consumption of specific food products.[219] For example, it has been reported that some soft drink marketers promote endorsements from celebrities with particular appeal to minority children, such as hip-hop artists.[220] Soft drink companies also are said to have used street marketing campaigns, sending teens into minority neighborhoods to give out free product samples. Food companies also have used sponsorships to promote brand awareness among minority communities. A panelist cited as an example the promotional campaign co-sponsored by a fast food company and a beverage company that distributed African- American history materials to children in schools.[221]

Another panelist discussed research currently underway about whether healthy lifestyle messages should be tailored to the race and socioeconomic status of the intended audience. The panelist explained that research indicates the messages parents want may vary by race and sometimes by socioeconomic status.[222] For example, some parents might want help with basic parenting skills, whereas others simply want nutrition guidance.[223] Some Hispanic mothers surveyed were unsure how many fruits and vegetables their children should eat daily or what limits on media usage they should be setting.[224] Some African-American mothers reported having difficulty negotiating food choices within the household, especially when an elder lived in the same household.[225] Based on the initial findings of the research, the panelist suggested that "one-size-fits-all" messages are likely not as effective as culturally tailored messages for specific racial/ethnic and socioeconomic groups.[226]

B. Food Industry Initiatives

Most of the product and packaging initiatives of the food industry taken in response to obesity concerns, as described in Section III, have been designed to appeal to the general population, rather than to specific minority populations. One reported exception is the reformulation of a General Mills product. The company had increased the soluble fiber content of its regular Cheerios cereal. It then reported observing that consumption of regular Cheerios was relatively low within the African-American community, while consumption of Honey Nut Cheerios was very high.[227] After increasing the soluble fiber content of Honey Nut Cheerios to match that of its regular Cheerios and marketing the reformulated product with health-promotion messages targeted to African-Americans, General Mills measured an increase in consumption of the reformulated product by 700,000 new households with children, including many African- American households.[228]

Given that much remains unknown about the differences between various racial and ethnic minority communities with respect to the impact of food marketing, one panelist suggested that the industry should use its access to data on market segmentation to develop strategic messaging and consumer education for different racial and socioeconomic groups.[229]

C. Media and Entertainment Industry Initiatives

Many workshop participants agreed that special attention must be paid to reaching parents and children from minority groups, given the disproportionate obesity rates of children in these communities.[230] In particular, some participants said that cultural differences within the African- American and Hispanic communities may call for different approaches with respect to media campaigns.[231] For example, Univision reported research suggesting that the media play a greater role as trusted source of information within the Hispanic community than they do within the general population.[232] Additionally, Univision said that it has conducted studies with Nielsen that indicate that over 50% of Hispanic viewers actually discuss commercials, as compared to only 6% of the non-Hispanic population.[233] This gives media catering to the Hispanic community a greater opportunity to empower their audiences with information.

Participants emphasized that there are some challenges to reaching certain minority groups through the media, however. One challenge is that only a limited number of networks specifically target minority audiences and the content directed at children on those networks is fairly limited. For example, BET, a major network catering to African-American audiences, does not feature programming intended for young children.[234] Another challenge mentioned by participants is that messages suited for mainstream audiences are not necessarily effective in reaching minority communities.

Some participants stated that a greater understanding of the cultural and environmental factors influencing the eating habits and physical activity of minority groups is needed and could lead to a more productive discussion about the media channels, types of programming, and message content that would work best to communicate health and wellness.[235] For example, as a few participants observed, factors such as access to fresh fruits and vegetables, grocery stores, and safe parks and neighborhoods in which to play, all have an impact on the health and wellness of some racial and ethnic communities.[236] One panelist suggested that, combined with fewer advertising signals to eat more nutritious foods, the relatively limited access to healthier foods in minority communities (due to fewer grocery stores and more fast food restaurants) may partially explain the higher obesity rates among African-American and Hispanic youth relative to non-Hispanic white youth.[237] Furthermore, other panelists commented that suggestions to get active and play might be less viable in urban communities where safety is a concern.

VI. SELF-REGULATORY STANDARDS FOR FOOD MARKETING TO CHILDREN

A. Value of Self-Regulatory Approach

A major goal of the workshop was to provide a forum for an examination of self- regulatory standards for responsible marketing of foods and beverages to children. Effective industry self-regulation can have significant benefits, and can, in many instances, address problems more quickly, creatively, and flexibly than government regulation.[238] For self- regulation to be effective, however, it should clearly address the problems it seeks to remedy, adjust to new developments within the industry, be enforced and widely followed by affected industry members, and be visible and accessible to the public. In addition, the self-regulatory body must be independent from its member firms to objectively measure their performance and impose sanctions for noncompliance. Self-regulation can be particularly beneficial in instances where it covers marketing activities that the FTC, FDA, and other agencies lack the authority to challenge. Self-regulation, for example, can address practices that are neither unfair nor deceptive under the FTC Act. It can also address such activities without raising significant First Amendment concerns that might be presented by government-imposed restrictions of truthful, non-misleading speech. The FTC and HHS generally believe that self-regulation can be a useful tool, as long as it is "carefully tailored" to the problem at hand and there is no anti-competitive effect.[239]

B. CARU Self-Regulatory Standards

1. Standards and Enforcement

A major focus of the discussion at the workshop was the Children's Advertising Review Unit ("CARU"), the principal industry self-regulatory group that governs advertising directed to children, including food advertising. The advertising industry created CARU in 1974, and CARU is directly funded by annual fees paid by companies who advertise to children.[240] CARU's policy and direction are set by the National Advertising Review Council ("NARC"), a group made up of the Council of Better Business Bureaus ("CBBB"), and the three major advertising associations – the Association of National Advertisers ("ANA"), the American Association of Advertising Agencies ("AAAA"), and the American Advertising Federation ("AAF").[241] The CBBB administers the day-to-day operation of CARU.

CARU's mandate is to ensure that all advertising targeted to children under the age of 12 is truthful, accurate, and takes into consideration young children's cognitive abilities. To achieve that mandate, NARC created the *Self-Regulatory Guidelines for Children's Advertising* ("CARU Guides"), a set of basic principles and guidelines that apply to child-directed advertising in all media.[242] (The CARU Guides are set forth in Appendix B.) The CARU Guides, among other things, seek to deter the use of techniques in advertising that might exploit a child or confuse a child about the value or benefit of a particular product and include principles that may go beyond just prohibiting deceptive or misleading advertising.

In many respects, the CARU Guides reflect general self-regulatory principles used by others. For example, GMA has its own set of self-regulatory principles for its food industry members that parallel many of the CARU Guides.[243] Television broadcast and cable network advertising clearance standards also impose similar standards.[244] And the International Chamber of Commerce ("ICC") incorporates, in its Code of Advertising Practices, many of the same approaches for encouraging responsible and non-deceptive industry advertising to children.[245] Finally, many individual companies have their own internal guidelines that govern how they advertise and market to children.[246]

Like most of these initiatives, the CARU Guides do not tell advertisers what foods they can and cannot market to children. Rather, they seek to prevent the use of techniques in advertising that might deceive or confuse children, or undermine the role of parents in selecting what products their children can have or purchase. For example, although the CARU Guides do not prohibit the advertising of "low-nutrition" or "snack foods," they do prohibit misleading children into thinking that a "low-nutrition" product is nutritious, or that a "snack food" could serve as a substitute for a meal.[247] They also prohibit ads that might encourage children to eat excessive amounts of foods or to pester their parents to buy them.[248] Although the CARU Guides do not limit the use of licensed characters or celebrities to sell foods or other products to children, they, like FCC regulations, do prohibit advertisers from using popular program personalities or characters to sell any product during or adjacent to the TV program in which they appear.[249] Other CARU Guides require that depictions of foods should encourage "sound use" of the product "with a view toward healthy development of the child and development of good nutritional practices," and that ads "representing mealtime should clearly and adequately depict the role of the product within the framework of a balanced diet."[250]

With a staff of six, CARU reports that it reviews roughly 1,000 commercials each month, in addition to print and radio ads and Web sites.[251] Its monitoring focuses on media "directed" to children under the age of 12. This includes programming on "Nickelodeon, Cartoon Network, and Radio Disney, broadcast and cable TV during traditional children's day parts and fringe and early prime time programming with a significant under-12 audience demographic."[252]

In its 30-year history, CARU has opened inquiries into more than 1,200 specific child- directed ads. According to a NARC report issued in May 2004,[253] about 150 of CARU's formal and informal inquiries[254] have concerned food advertising (although in the last few years many of those inquiries have not directly concerned claims in food ads but rather data collection and children's privacy issues on food company websites).[255] In virtually all instances, the advertiser complied or ended the specific advertising campaign, often indicating that it would take into account CARU's concerns in future campaigns.

Companies found to have violated the CARU Guides are identified in a CARU press release and their violation (if they refuse to change a potentially deceptive ad) can be referred to the FTC.[256] CARU does not fine or otherwise penalize violators, including repeat violators.[257]

Over the years, NARC has changed the CARU Guides in response to new advertising techniques or issues.[258] For example, a major revision in 1996 added a new section addressing children's privacy and data collection on the Internet. In addition, NARC was considering other changes to the CARU Guides and to CARU itself in the weeks leading up to the workshop.

2. Analysis of Self-Regulation

In the panel discussions and in the comments received for the workshop, views on the value of the CARU Guides varied widely. Overall, industry members felt the guides have "worked well" and have done an adequate job in protecting children from false, misleading, or inappropriate food ads. Consumer group participants were far less enthusiastic about the guides, indicating that self-regulation was "not working,"[259] was a "failure,"[260] or should be "abandoned."[261] Senator Harkin, who offered opening remarks at the workshop, expressed the view that self-regulation to date has not been effective.[262] Some participants pointed to recent ad campaigns that they say violated the CARU Guides, arguing that CARU, whose budget is funded by those it regulates, cannot be relied on to independently police food industry advertising.[263]

A key topic of discussion was whether the CARU Guides, themselves, need updating to reflect today's marketing. One participant, representing a consumer advocacy group, was concerned that the guides do not address some of the "newer forms of advertising and marketing such as in-school advertising, advergaming, and peer-to-peer marketing."[264] By just covering national advertising, according to another participant, the CARU Guides do not reach new forms of promotion in today's marketplace such as use of interactive technology to market products targeted to children.[265] The discussion of the CARU Guides at the workshop also focused on issues not directly related to their scope, such as the size of the staff available to administer the guides; the visibility of CARU to the public and, in particular, to parents; and the limited sanctions available for companies who violate the guides.

In response to many of these concerns, GMA put forward a proposal to strengthen CARU. (The GMA Proposal is set forth in Appendix C.) It asked that NARC revise the CARU Guides to "address" advertising contained in electronic games and interactive websites, and to ensure that third-party licensed characters are used "appropriately" in advertising.[266] The GMA proposal did not set out how the guides should limit ads in electronic games or interactive websites or what would be an appropriate use of licensed characters, leaving it to NARC to develop specific restrictions it believes would be appropriate. GMA also recommended that the CARU Guides prohibit paid product placement on children's television programming, although the FCC requirement of a buffer between program content and commercial content during children's programming on cable and broadcast television already effectively prohibits such placements.[267]

GMA's proposal addressed other criticisms of the current CARU program. For example, GMA recommended that: CARU's staff be "substantially" increased; parents be given immediate and direct access to CARU to express concerns about advertising directed to children through mechanisms such as a toll-free complaint line; and CARU's decisions be easily available on the CARU website.[268] GMA also asked that CARU strengthen its program to pre-screen ads and expand its advisory board to bring in experts on nutrition and health. GMA's proposal, however, did not address one of the key complaints about the CARU process, namely the limited sanctions available for violators of the guides.[269]

One industry member described the GMA proposal as a "good start."[270] One consumer group, however, criticized the proposal, because it was sponsored by only nine out of 140 companies in the trade association.[271] In addition, although the proposal was commended for expanding the CARU guides to cover some other forms of advertising, it was deemed deficient by the consumer group for its failure to grant CARU jurisdiction over advertising and promotions in schools.[272]

Following the workshop, NARC began to consider GMA's recommendations. In a letter sent to the FTC on September 15, 2005, NARC announced several revisions to CARU that partially adopted GMA's suggestions. (The NARC letter is set forth in Appendix D.) NARC stated, for example, that CARU has set up an online consumer complaint form on its website, would expand its voluntary pre-review system for children's ads, and would add additional members who have expertise in children's health to its advisory board. NARC also committed to providing annual briefings to the FTC and HHS.

NARC has indicated that it is still looking at several other changes suggested by GMA. For example, it has directed CARU to look at ways to monitor advertising placed in electronic games; it is waiting for a report from CARU on interactive online games; it has set up a task force to examine product placement; and it has asked CARU to contact interested parties to assess what might be done regarding the use of third-party licensing of characters. The NARC letter did not indicate whether it was planning to expand the size of the CARU staff and its budget, as suggested by GMA.

In addition, NARC and CBBB recently announced the formation of a new self-regulatory working group that will be reviewing the CARU Guides in their entirety to make sure that they reflect the changing environment and the full range of marketing issues that have developed in recent years, including concerns about childhood obesity.[273] The working group will evaluate the use of new forms of marketing (such as the Internet), product placement, and cartoon characters to market foods to children. It also will explore a broad range of other ideas as to how self- regulatory standards for food marketing to kids could be modified.

The CBBB/CARU self-regulatory working group commenced its work in March 2006. The CBBB/CARU working group reports that it has solicited participation from a wide range of food industry members, academics, consumer advocates, and public health groups to develop proposals to modify the CARU Guides. According to the CBBB/CARU working group, it will make specific recommendations for changes to the Guides, will seek input from the public on these recommendations, and, after considering such information, NARC will announce any changes that it has decided to make to the CARU Guides and the enforcement process.

At the workshop, there was much discussion about whether the CARU Guides should include nutritional standards for foods marketed to children. In January 2005, the Center for Science in the Public Interest ("CSPI") called for a new set of guidelines that would change how foods and beverages are promoted to children by directly taking on the "good food/bad food" debate.[274] CSPI's proposed *Guidelines for Responsible Food Marketing to Children* ("CSPI

Proposal") would restructure the existing self-regulatory system by setting specific nutritional thresholds that foods and beverages would have to meet before they could be marketed to children under the age of 18. In addition, the CSPI Proposal would prohibit the use of certain marketing techniques, such as licensed characters and premiums, for foods that, under those thresholds, were of "poor nutrition quality."[275]

The CSPI Proposal would effectively limit the types of foods advertised to children.

Under the CSPI proposal, many soft drinks, caffeinated drinks, sports drinks, sugared breakfast cereals, snack foods, and quick-service restaurant foods could not be marketed to children.[276] In its comment for the workshop, CARU indicated that imposing such restrictions is not a part of CARU's mandate.[277] Nonetheless, some participants contended that if CARU continues to focus on how foods are marketed, rather than on what foods are marketed, self-regulation would do little to change children's diets. The representative from CSPI stated, "simply changing the way a sales pitch is couched is often irrelevant, because the real problem is that the food itself undermines children's diets and health."[278]

In questioning the reasonableness and practicality of the CSPI Proposal, an industry official asked who would set the nutritional standards and how would they be applied to the widely varying products food companies sell.[279] CARU asserted in its comment that food products are not inherently dangerous or inappropriate – all foods may be safely incorporated into a balanced diet, so it follows that companies should not be held to a standard that prohibits some foods from being marketed.[280] Other industry participants were concerned that imposing such standards for all foods would be unworkable, because many foods could never meet those standards.

CSPI stated that existing models can be used to come up with self-regulatory nutritional standards.[281] Others acknowledged that developing such standards would be difficult but believed it should be tried,[282] although another participant expressed distrust of industry implementing nutritional guidelines and urged that government enforce them.[283] A representative from the European Union noted that, as a practical matter, even those who would prefer government standards of enforcement should support expanded self-regulatory efforts, given that self-regulation is likely to have an effect long before any government statute or regulation could be implemented.[284]

In sum, the workshop record illustrates widely divergent views and many unanswered questions on the merits and difficulties of developing nutritional standards for food products marketed to children.

VII. CONCLUSION AND RECOMMENDATIONS

The record developed at the workshop indicates that members of the food industry and the media are taking steps to address childhood obesity. They also have instituted a variety of promising initiatives that use the power of the marketplace to encourage children to eat better and exercise more. Although there are questions regarding whether these industry efforts go far enough, the FTC and HHS are encouraged by the progress being made.

The agencies also are encouraged by the discussions (some only preliminary) concerning the ways in which industry self-regulation can be improved. Several participants acknowledged at the close of the workshop that the process of expanding and enhancing self-regulation will require a sustained effort and that it is important that there be a continuing dialogue on how best to move the process forward.[285] One approach would be to convene a formal dialogue, conducted under the auspices of a third-party facilitator, with broad participation by all stakeholders. The agencies were considering such an approach when NARC and CBBB announced the formation of the CBBB/CARU working group effort to review and propose changes to the CARU Guides.

The agencies have concluded that the CBBB/CARU working group should be given a reasonable amount of time to complete its review and develop and implement changes to the CARU Guides before determining whether to recommend other alternatives. The agencies recognize that broad industry support is important to the ultimate success of any self-regulatory changes, and there appears to be such support for the CBBB/CARU working group. In addition, because NARC seems to have the ability to expeditiously adopt and implement changes to the CARU Guides, the CBBB/CARU working group may lead to changes sooner than other alternatives. Finally, the CBBB/CARU working group appears to provide a reasonable opportunity for consumer advocates, public health groups, and other stakeholders to participate in its process. To encourage participation and ultimate acceptance of its resolution of contested issues, the agencies underscore that the CBBB/CARU working group should establish and employ a process that is as open and transparent as possible.

The FTC and HHS emphasize that the government's follow-up report discussed below will closely evaluate the changes that the NARC Board makes to the self-regulatory process, including assessing whether these changes satisfactorily address the specific recommendations for self-regulation set forth below in this chapter, or whether additional steps are necessary.

Building on the initiatives highlighted at the workshop, the agencies recommend:

Industry Self-Regulation of Food Marketing to Children

General Process of Self-Regulation: The following steps should be taken as soon as practicable to improve the CARU process:

- NARC should expand CARU's advisory board to include individuals with more diverse experience, such as nutrition, child health, and developmental psychology experts.
- NARC should evaluate and determine whether CARU' s staff and resources are sufficient to monitor and enforce adequately the CARU Guides. This determination should be made in light of any changes made in response to the recommendations of this chapter, and then be revisited in light of any further changes made in response to the CBBB/CARU working group.
- CARU should make it easier for parents and others to file complaints, and its decisions should be made more readily available and accessible to the public online.

Broader Issues of Self-Regulation of Food Marketing to Children: Industry also needs to consider a wide range of additional options as to how self-regulation could be modified to assist in combating childhood obesity. Among other things, the agencies recommend that the issues addressed include:

- how to modify the CARU Guides to address forms of marketing foods to children other than traditional advertising.[286]
- whether it would be beneficial and practicable to modify the CARU Guides to include (or to develop a new set of guides that would identify) minimum nutritional standards for foods that are marketed to children, standards that shift marketing to children to focus on more nutritious, lower-calorie foods, or other measures that would improve the overall nutritional profile of foods marketed to children, recognizing that the appropriate standards or measures may vary based on product category.
- the feasibility of an independent non-profit or public health organization developing a seal or logo program which identifies more nutritious, lower-calorie foods.
- to what extent paid product placement of foods in contexts other than television programming (e.g., movies, video games, websites) is appropriate.

- what additional sanctions or other measures should be incorporated into the CARU Guides to deter violations, especially repeated violations.

Food Company Initiatives

- *Products:* Food companies should continue and expand their efforts to create new products and reformulate products, especially those marketed to children, to make them lower in calories and more nutritious. Companies should also increase their efforts to make nutritious, lower-calorie products appealing to children and more convenient for them to consume.
- *Packaging:* Food companies should continue and expand their use of packaging, such as smaller portion, single-serving, and other packaging cues, to help consumers, including children, control portion size and calories. Companies should also increase their efforts to package nutritious, lower-calorie products in ways that are more appealing to children and more convenient for parents to prepare.
- *Labeling:* Food companies should explore the effectiveness of labeling initiatives, such as nutrition icons and seal programs, in helping consumers easily identify nutritious, lower-calorie products. Food companies should conduct consumer research to ensure that such initiatives do not mislead consumers and to identify the techniques that most clearly and effectively convey nutrition and calorie information.
- *Advertising/Marketing:* Food companies should review and revise their marketing activities to improve the overall nutritional profile of the products they market to children. Recognizing that appropriate standards or measures may vary based on company or product category, the agencies recommend that companies consider adopting: (1) minimum nutritional standards for the foods they market to children; or (2) standards that shift their marketing to children to emphasize more their nutritious, lower-calorie products; or (3) other measures that help to improve the overall nutritional profile of the products they market to children.
- Food companies should also continue to explore ways to improve public education efforts. Consumer research on the efficacy of various fitness and nutrition messages in marketing to children will help to identify simple and effective messages.

- *Marketing and Sales in Schools:* In addition to the wellness policies developed by local schools, food companies should review and revise their policies and practices to improve the overall nutritional profile of the products they market and sell to children in schools. The agencies recognize that the appropriate standards or measures may vary based on product category.

Media/Entertainment Company Initiatives

- *Educational Messages:* The media and entertainment companies should continue to explore ways to improve their efforts to disseminate, and to work with others to disseminate, clear and effective educational messages to children and parents about nutrition and fitness, including incorporating such messages into programming.
- *Character Licensing:* The media and entertainment companies should review and revise their practices to foster the licensing of children's television and movie characters for use with more nutritious, lower-calorie products.

Public Education Campaigns/Community Outreach

- Food companies, advertising agencies, the media, entertainment companies, academic institutions, and others should expand their efforts jointly to develop and support substantial public education programs that promote nutrition and fitness to children, including outreach programs in local communities. These programs should use simple, positive, consistent messages that have been tested for effectiveness and are repeated across various platforms and venues to increase their impact.

Marketing of Foods to Racial and Ethnic Communities

- Food companies should include in their overall marketing strategy efforts to promote more nutritious, lower-calorie products to racial and ethnic minority populations in which childhood obesity rates are high.

- •Food companies, the media, and entertainment companies should also tailor their public education programs and other outreach efforts to promote better nutrition and fitness in racial and ethnic minority populations in which childhood obesity rates are high.

The FTC and HHS hope that the momentum created by the workshop will drive an expansion of food and media industry efforts to address childhood obesity, both through individual company initiatives and through a strengthened industry-wide self-regulatory system. The agencies will monitor closely future developments in food marketing to children. After allowing time for the private sector to consider and respond to the recommendations in this chapter, one or both of the agencies will issue a follow-up report assessing the extent to which positive, concrete measures have been implemented and identifying what, if any, additional steps may be warranted to ensure adequate progress is being made to address childhood obesity.

APPENDIX A. WORKSHOP AGENDA AND LIST OF PANELISTS/PARTICIPANTS

July 14-15, 2005

Day One:

8:00 AM	*Registration*
9:00 AM	*Welcome and Introduction*
	Keynote Remarks
	Chairman Deborah Platt Majoras. Federal Trade Commission
	Dr. Lester Crawford. Acting Commissioner, Food and Drug Administration
9:30 AM	*Congressional Remarks*
	Senator Tom Harkin (Iowa)
9:45 AM	*Presentation: Overview of Health Risks with Childhood Obesity and the* Research Concerning the Factors Related to Childhood Obesity
	Dr. William Dietz

	Director, Division of Nutrition and Physical Activity, CDC, HHS
10:15 AM	*Presentation: Ongoing FTC Staff Research Concerning Food Advertising to Children on Television*
	Dr. Pauline M. Ippolito
	Associate Director, Bureau of Economics, FTC
10:30 AM	Break
10:45 AM	*Panel 1: The Past, Present, and Future of Marketing of Foods to Children*

Moderators: Thomas B. Pahl. Assistant Director for
Advertising Practices, FTC
Dr. Van S. Hubbard. Director, Division of
Nutrition Research Coordination, NIH, HHS

Panelists:

- Dr. Nancy M. Childs, Professor of Food Marketing, St. Joseph's University
- Brady Darvin, Senior Director, Strottman International
- Dr. Sonya A. Grier, Robert Wood Johnson Health & Society Scholar, University of Pennsylvania
- Jeffrey McIntyre, Senior Legislative and Federal Affairs Officer, American Psychological Association
- Dr. Elizabeth S. Moore, Associate Professor of Marketing, University of Notre Dame
- Dick O'Brien, Executive Vice President, Director of Government Relations, American Association of Advertising Agencies

12:00 noon	*Questions from the Audience*
12:15 PM	*Lunch Break*
1:15 PM	*Remarks*
	Commissioner Pamela Jones Harbour Federal Trade Commission
1:30 PM	*Panel 2-A: Current Industry Efforts to Market Foods to Help Improve Children's Health, Including Changes in Products and Packaging*

Moderators: Maureen Ohlhausen. Director, Office of Policy
Planning, FTC

Panelists:

- Michael Donahue, Vice President, U.S. Communications and Customer Satisfaction, McDonald's USA
- Bob Goldin, Executive Vice President, Technomic, Inc.
- Kendall J. Powell, Executive Vice President and COO, U.S. Retail, General Mills
- Dr. Rebecca S. Reeves, President, American Dietetic Association
- Abigail L. Rodgers, Vice President of Wellness Strategies and Communication, The Coca-Cola Company
- Dr. Lisa Sutherland, Research Assistant Professor, University of North Carolina

2:30 PM   Questions from the Audience

2:45 PM   *Panel 2-B: Current Industry Efforts to Market Foods to Help Improve Children's Health, Including Changes in Advertising and Marketing*

　　　　　Moderators: Michelle K. Rusk. Senior Attorney, FTC
　　　　　　　　　　　Dr. Howard Zucker. Deputy Assistant Secretary for Health, HHS

　　　Panelists:

- Dr. Daniel S. Acuff, Co-Founder and Director, YMS Consulting
- Mark H. Berlind, Executive Vice President, Global Corporate Affairs, Kraft Foods
- Linda Brugler, Nutrition Marketing Manager, Produce for Better Health Foundation
- Dr. Carol Byrd-Bredbenner, Professor of Nutrition and Extension Specialist, Rutgers University
- Alan Harris, Executive Vice President, Chief Marketing and Customer Officer, Kellogg Company
- Brock Leach, Senior Vice President, New Growth Platforms, and Chief Innovation Officer, PepsiCo, Inc.
- Bob McKinnon, Founder and President, YELLOWBRICKROAD Communications

3:45 PM   *Questions from the Audience*

4:00 PM   *Break*

        Moderators: Rielle C. Montague. Attorney, FTC

                Dr. Elizabeth Edgerton. Director of Clinical Prevention, AHRQ, HHS

        Panelists:

- Heidi Arthur, Senior Vice President, Group Campaign Director, The Advertising Council
- Jorge Daboub, Vice President of Marketing and Business Development, Univision Television Group
- Ivan J. Juzang, Founder and President, MEE Productions
- Dr. Jennifer Kotler, Director for Knowledge Management, Department of Education and Research, Sesame Workshop
- Victoria Rideout, Vice President, Kaiser Family Foundation
- Marva Smalls, Executive Vice President of Public Affairs and Chief of Staff, Nickelodeon Networks

5:15 PM   *Questions from the Audience*

5:30 PM   *Open Forum*

6:00 PM   *Adjourn for the Day*

Day Two:

8:00 AM   *Registration*

8:30 AM   *Remarks*

        Vice Admiral Richard H. Carmona Surgeon General

        Commissioner Thomas B. Leary Federal Trade Commission

9:00 AM   *Panel 4: Current Self-Regulatory and Other Standards for Marketing Food to Children*

        Moderators: Richard F. Kelly. Senior Attorney, FTC

                Dr. Barbara Schneeman. Director, Office of Nutritional Products, Labeling, and Dietary Supplements, CF SAN, FDA, HHS

        Panelists:

- Charlotte Hebebrand, Food Safety, Health and Consumer Affairs Section, European Commission Delegation
- Elizabeth L. Lascoutx, Director, Children's Advertising Review Unit
- Patti Miller, Vice President and Director of the Children & the Media Program, Children Now
- Dr. Kathryn Montgomery, Professor of Communication, American University
- Wally Snyder, President and CEO, American Advertising Federation
- Dr. Margo Wootan, Director of Nutrition Policy, Center for Science in the Public Interest

10:15 AM   *Questions from the Audience*

10:30 AM   *Open Forum*

11:00 AM   *Break*

11:15 AM   *Panel 5:* Next Steps – What Should the Government and the Private Sector Do to Help Make Children's Diets Healthier and Encourage Responsible Marketing

Moderators: Mary K. Engle
Associate Director for Advertising Practices, FTC
Dr. Michael O'Grady
Assistant Secretary for Planning and Evaluation, HHS

Presentation: Overview of the Institute of Medicine Studies Addressing the Marketing of Food & Beverages to Children
Vivica Kraak. Senior Program Officer, Food and Nutrition Board, IOM

Panelists:

- Mark H. Berlind, Executive Vice President, Global Corporate Affairs, Kraft Foods
- Dan Jaffe, Executive Vice President, Association of National Advertisers
- Dr. Penny Kris-Etherton, Nutrition Committee, American Heart Association

- Brock Leach, Senior Vice President, New Growth Platforms, and Chief Innovation Officer, PepsiCo, Inc.
- C. Manly Molpus, President and CEO, Grocery Manufacturers of America
- Dr. Susan Linn, Associate Director of the Media Center, Judge Baker Children's Center and Harvard Medical School
- Dr. Donald Lee Shifrin, Task Force on Obesity, American Academy of Pediatrics

12:45 PM   *Closing Remarks*

Dr. Michael O'Grady. Assistant Secretary for Planning and Evaluation, HHS

Lydia B. Parnes. Director, Bureau of Consumer Protection, FTC

Please Note: Due to space constraints, persons will be admitted to the FTC Conference Center, 601 New Jersey Avenue, N.W., on a first-come, first-served basis beginning at 8:00 AM on each day of the workshop. Pre-registration does not guarantee that space will be available. Workshop attendees may not save seats for others. Overflow seating will be available at the FTC Headquarters Building, 600 Pennsylvania Avenue, N.W.

Workshop attendees must undergo security screening each time they enter the building, and will need to show a valid form of photo identification, such as a driver's license.

The FTC Conference Center is accessible to people with disabilities. If you need an accommodation related to a disability, please call Todd Dickey at 202-326-3648

APPENDIX B.
SELF-REGULATORY GUIDELINES
FOR CHILDREN'S ADVERTISING[1]

The Children's Advertising Review Unit (CARU) of the Council of Better Business Bureaus was established in 1974 by the National Advertising Review Council (NARC) to promote responsible children's advertising and to respond to public concerns. The NARC is a strategic alliance of the advertising industry and the Council of Better Business Bureaus (CBBB). The NARC's Board of Directors comprises key executives from the CBBB, the American Association of Advertising Agencies (AAAA), the American Advertising Federation (AAF) and the Association of National Advertisers (ANA). The NARC Board sets policy for CARU's self-regulatory program, which is administered by the CBBB and is funded directly by members of the children's advertising industry.

CARU's Academic and Business Advisory Boards provide guidance on general issues concerning children's advertising. The Academic Advisory Board, composed of leading experts in education, communication, child development, child mental health and nutrition, consults on individual issues and cases, and assists in the review of the Guidelines. The Business Advisory Board, composed of prominent industry leaders, provides guidance in marketing and advertising trends and practices and also assists in the review of the Guidelines.

CARU's basic activities are the review and evaluation of child-directed advertising in all media, and online privacy practices as they affect children. When these are found to be misleading, inaccurate or inconsistent with the Guidelines, CARU seeks changes through the voluntary cooperation of advertisers and Website operators.

---

[1] Children's Advertising Review Unit. Council of Better Business Bureaus, Inc. 70 West 36th Street, New York, NY 10018.

The Children's Advertising Guidelines have been in existence since 1972 when they were published by the Association of National Advertisers, Inc. to encourage truthful and accurate advertising sensitive to the special nature of children. Subsequently, the advertising community established CARU to serve as an independent manager of the industry's self-regulatory program. CARU edited and republished the Self-Regulatory Guidelines for Children's Advertising in 1975, revising them periodically to address changes in the marketing and media landscapes. A major revision in 1996 added a new section addressing children's privacy and data collection on the Internet. The assistance of CARU's Advisory Board, and of other children's advertisers, their agencies and trade associations has been invaluable.

Copyright 1975, 2003. Council of Better Business Bureaus, Inc. The name Children's Advertising Review Unit is a registered service mark of the Council of Better Business Bureaus, Inc. Seventh Edition 2003.

Generally CARU reviews advertising in all media directed to children under 12 years of age. To harmonize with the federal Children's Online Privacy Protection Act of 1998 (COPPA) CARU reviews online privacy practices involving children under 13 years of age.

CARU provides a general advisory service for advertisers and agencies and also is a source of informational material for children, parents and educators. CARU encourages advertisers to develop and promote the dissemination of educational messages to children consistent with the Children's Television Act of 1990.

Principles

Seven basic Principles underlie CARU's Guidelines for advertising directed to children under 12:

1. Advertisers should always take into account the level of knowledge, sophistication and maturity of the audience to which their message is primarily directed. Yo unger children have a limited capacity for evaluating the credibility of information they receive. They also may lack the ability to understand the nature of the personal information they disclose on the Internet. Advertisers, therefore, have a special responsibility to protect children from their own susceptibilities.
2. Realizing that children are imaginative and that make-believe play constitutes an important part of the growing up process, advertisers should exercise care not to exploit unfairly the imaginative quality of children. Unreasonable expectations of product quality or performance should not be stimulated either directly or indirectly by advertising.
3. Products and content which are inappropriate for children should not be advertised or promoted directly to children.
4. Recognizing that advertising may play an important part in educating the child, advertisers should communicate information in a truthful and accurate manner and in language understandable to young children with full recognition that the child may learn practices from advertising which can affect his or her health and well-being.
5. Advertisers are urged to capitalize on the potential of advertising to influence behavior by developing advertising that, wherever possible, addresses itself to positive and beneficial social behavior, such as friendship, kindness, honesty, justice, generosity and respect for others.

6. Care should be taken to incorporate minority and other groups in advertisements in order to present positive and pro-social roles and role models wherever possible. Social stereotyping and appeals to prejudice should be avoided.

7. Although many influences affect a child's personal and social development, it remains the prime responsibility of the parents to provide guidance for children. Advertisers should contribute to this parent-child relationship in a constructive manner.

These Principles embody the philosophy upon which CARU's mandate is based. The Principles, and not the Guidelines themselves, determine the scope of our review. The Guidelines effectively anticipate and address many of the areas requiring scrutiny in child-directed advertising, but they are illustrative rather than limiting. Where no specific Guideline addresses the issues of concern to CARU, it is these broader Principles that CARU applies in evaluating advertising directed to the uniquely impressionable and vulnerable child audience.

Interpretation of the Guidelines

Because children are in the process of developing their knowledge of the physical and social world they are more limited than adults in the experience and skills required to evaluate advertising and to make purchase decisions. For these reasons, certain presentations and techniques which may be appropriate for adult-directed advertising may mislead children if used in child-directed advertising.

The function of the Guidelines is to delineate those areas that need particular attention to help avoid deceptive advertising messages to children. The intent is to help advertisers deal sensitively and honestly with children and is not meant to deprive them, or children, of the benefits of innovative advertising approaches.

The Guidelines have been kept general in the belief that responsible advertising comes in many forms and that diversity should be encouraged. The goal in all cases should be to fulfill the spirit as well as the letter of the Guidelines and of the Principles on which they are based.

Scope of the Guidelines

The Guidelines apply to advertising addressed to children under twelve years of age in all media, including print, broadcast and cable television, radio, video, point-of-sale and online advertising and packaging. CARU interprets this as including fundraising activities and sponsor identifications on non-commercial television and radio. One section applies to adult-directed advertising only when a potential child-safety concern exists (see Safety, below). Another section addresses children's online privacy (see Interactive Electronic Media).

Product Presentations and Claims

Children look at, listen to and remember many different elements in advertising. Therefore, advertisers need to examine the total advertising message to be certain that the net communication will not mislead or misinform children.

1. Copy, sound and visual presentations should not mislead children about product or performance characteristics. Such characteristics may include, but are not limited to, size, speed, method of operation, color, sound, durability and nutritional benefits.
2. The advertising presentation should not mislead children about benefits from use of the product. Such benefits may include, but are not limited to, the acquisition of strength, status, popularity, growth, proficiency and intelligence.
3. Care should be taken not to exploit a child's imagination. Fantasy, including animation, is appropriate for younger as well as older children. However, it should not create unattainable performance expectations nor exploit the younger child's difficulty in distinguishing between the real and the fanciful.
4. The performance and use of a product should be demonstrated in a way that can be duplicated by the child for whom the product is intended.
5. Products should be shown used in safe ways, in safe environments and in safe situations.
6. What is included and excluded in the initial purchase should be clearly established.
7. The amount of product featured should be within reasonable levels for the situation depicted.
8. Representation of food products should be made so as to encourage sound use of the product with a view toward healthy development of the child and development of good nutritional practices.
9. Advertisements representing mealtime should clearly and adequately depict the role of the product within the framework of a balanced diet.

10. Snack foods should be clearly represented as such, and not as substitutes for meals.
11. In advertising videos, films and interactive software, advertisers should take care that only those which are age-appropriate are advertised to children. If an industry rating system is available, the rating label should be prominently displayed. Inconsistencies will be brought to the attention of the rating entity.
12. Portrayals or encouragement of behavior inappropriate for children (e.g.: violence or sexuality) and presentations that could frighten or provoke anxiety in children should be avoided.
13. If objective claims are made in an advertisement directed to children, the advertiser should be able to supply adequate substantiation.

Sales Pressure

Children are not as prepared as adults to make judicious, independent purchase decisions Therefore, advertisers should avoid using extreme sales pressure in advertising presentations to children.

1. Children should not be urged to ask parents or others to buy products. Advertisements should not suggest that a parent or adult who purchases a product or service for a child is better, more intelligent or more generous than one who does not. Advertising directed toward children should not create a sense of urgency or exclusivity, for example, by using words like "now" and "only".
2. Benefits attributed to the product or service should be inherent in its use. Advertisements should not convey the impression that possession of a product will result in more acceptance of a child by his or her peers. Conversely, it should not be implied that lack of a product will cause a child to be less accepted by his or her peers. Advertisements should not imply that purchase and use of a product will confer upon the user the prestige, skills or other special qualities of characters appearing in advertising.
3. All price representations should be clearly and concisely set forth. Price minimizations such as "only" or "just" should not be used.

Disclosures and Disclaimers

Children have a more limited vocabulary and less developed language skills than do adolescents and adults. They read less well, if at all, and rely more on information presented pictorially than verbally. Simplified wording, such as "You have to put it together" instead of "Assembly required," significantly increases comprehension.

1. All disclosures and disclaimers that are material to a child should be in language understandable by the child audience, legible and prominent. When technology permits, both audio and video disclosures are encouraged, as is the use of demonstrative disclosures.
2. Advertising for unassembled products should clearly indicate that they need to be put together to be used properly.
3. If any item essential to use of the product, such as batteries, is not included, this fact should be disclosed clearly.
4. Information about products purchased separately, such as accessories or individual items in a collection, should be disclosed clearly.
5. If television advertising to children involves the use of a toll-free telephone number, it must be clearly stated, in both audio and video disclosures, that the child must get an adult's permission to call.
    a. In print or online advertising, this disclosure must be clearly and prominently displayed.
    b. In radio advertising, the audio disclosure must be clearly audible.
6. If an advertiser creates or sponsors an area in cyberspace, either through an online service or a Website, the name of the sponsoring company and/or brand should be prominently featured, (including, but not limited to wording such as "The ... Playground", or "Sponsored by ...").
7. If videotapes, CD-ROMs, DVDs or software marketed to children contain advertising or promotions (e.g. trailers) this fact should be clearly disclosed on the packaging, and the advertising itself should be separated from the program and clearly designated as advertising.

Comparative Claims

Advertising which compares the advertised product to another product may be difficult for young children to understand and evaluate. Comparative claims should be based on real product advantages that are understandable to the child audience.

1. Comparative advertising should provide factual information. Comparisons should not falsely represent other products or previous versions of the same product.
2. Comparative claims should be presented in ways that children understand clearly.
3. Comparative claims should be supported by appropriate and adequate substantiation.

Endorsement and Promotion by Program or Editorial Characters

Studies have shown that the mere appearance of a character with a product can significantly alter a child's perception of the product. Advertising presentations by program/editorial characters may hamper a young child's ability to distinguish between program/editorial content and advertising.

1. All personal endorsements should reflect the actual experiences and beliefs of the endorser. Celebrities and real-life authority figures may be used as product endorsers, presenters, or testifiers. However, extra care should be taken to avoid creating any false impression that the use of the product enhanced the celebrity's performance.
2. An endorser represented, either directly or indirectly, as an expert must possess qualifications appropriate to the particular expertise depicted in the endorsement.
3. Program personalities, live or animated, should not be used to sell products, premiums or services in or adjacent to programs primarily directed to children in which the same personality or character appears.
4. Products derived from or associated with program content primarily directed to children should not be advertised during or adjacent to that program.
5. In print media primarily designed for children, a character or personality associated with the editorial content of a publication should not be used to sell products, premiums or services in the same publication.
6. For print and interactive electronic media in which a product, service, or product/service-personality is featured in the editorial content (e.g., character- driven magazines or Websites, product-driven magazines or

Websites, and club newsletters) guideline 4 does not specifically apply. In these instances advertising content should nonetheless be clearly identified as such.

Premiums, Promotions and Sweepstakes

The use of premiums, promotions and sweepstakes in advertising has the potential to enhance the appeal of a product to a child. Therefore, special attention should be paid to the advertising of these marketing techniques to guard against exploiting children's immaturity.

Premiums

1. Children have difficulty distinguishing product from premium. If product advertising contains a premium message, care should be taken that the child's attention is focused primarily on the product. The premium message should be clearly secondary.
2. Conditions of a premium offer should be stated simply and clearly. "Mandatory" statements and disclosures should be stated in terms that can be understood by the child audience.

Kids' Clubs

In advertising to children, care should be taken not to mislead them into thinking they are joining a club when they are merely making a purchase or receiving a premium. Before an advertiser uses the word "club", certain minimum requirements should be met. These are:

1. Interactivity - The child should perform some act constituting an intentional joining of the club, and receive something in return. Merely watching a television program or eating in a particular restaurant, for example, does not constitute membership in a club.
2. Continuity - There should be an ongoing relationship between the club and the child member, for example, in the form of newsletter or activities, at regular intervals.

3. Exclusivity - The activities or benefits derived from membership in the club should be exclusive to its members, and not merely the result of purchasing a particular product.

Please see the Data Collection section of the Guidelines for Interactive Electronic Media for special considerations when fulfilling these requirements in the interactive media.

Sweepstakes and Contests

In advertising sweepstakes to children, care should be taken not to produce unrealistic expectations of the chances of winning, or inflated expectations of the prize(s) to be won. Therefore:

1. The prize(s) should be clearly depicted.
2. The likelihood of winning should be clearly disclosed in language clearly understandable to the child audience (for instance, where appropriate, "Many will enter, a few will win"). In appropriate media, disclosures must be included in the audio portion.
3. All prizes should be appropriate to the child audience.
4. Alternate means of entry should be disclosed.
5. Online contests or sweepstakes should not require the child to provide more information than is reasonably necessary. Any information collection must meet the requirements of the Data Collection section of the Guidelines and the federal Children's Online Privacy Protection Act (COPPA). [For examples of compliant information collection practices for this purpose, please visit <http://www.caru.org/news/ commentary.asp>].

Safety

Imitation, exploration and experimentation are important activities to children. They are attracted to commercials in general and may imitate product demonstrations and other actions without regard to risk. Many childhood accidents and injuries occur in the home, often involving abuse or misuse of common household products.

1. Products inappropriate for use by children should not be advertised directly to children. This is especially true for products labeled, "Keep out of the reach of children." Such inappropriate products or promotions include displaying or knowingly linking to the URL of a Website not in compliance with CARU's Guidelines. Additionally, such products should not be promoted directly to children by premiums or other means. Medications, drugs and supplemental vitamins should not be advertised to children.
2. Advertisements for children's products should show them being used by children in the appropriate age range. For instance, young children should not be shown playing with toys safe only for older children.
3. Adults should be shown supervising children when products or activities could involve a safety risk.
4. Advertisements should not portray adults or children in unsafe situations, or in acts harmful to themselves or others. For example, when athletic activities (such as bicycle riding or skateboarding) are shown, proper precautions and safety equipment should be depicted.
5. Advertisements should avoid demonstrations that encourage dangerous or inappropriate use or misuse of the product. This is particularly important when the demonstration can be easily reproduced by children and features products accessible to them.

Interactive Electronic Media

The guidelines contained in this section highlight issues unique to Internet and online advertising to children under 13. They are to be read within the broader context of the overall Guidelines, which apply to advertising in all media. For these purposes, the term "advertisers" also refers to any person who operates a commercial Website located on the Internet or an online service. Although all other sections of CARU's Self-Regulatory Guidelines for Children's Advertising address advertising directed to children under 12 years of age, in order to harmonize with the Federal Trade Commission's ("FTC") final rule implementing the Children's Online Privacy Protection Act of 1998 ("the Rule"), the guidelines contained in the section on Data Collection below apply to Websites directed to children under 13 years of age.

Just as these new media are rapidly evolving, so in all likelihood will this section of the Guidelines. Advances in technology, increased understanding of children's use of the medium, and the means by which these current guidelines are implemented will all contribute to the evolution of the "Interactive Electronic Media" section. CARU's aim is that the Guidelines will always support "notice", "choice" and "consent" as defined by the FTC, and reflect the latest developments in technology and its application to children's advertising.

Further, these children's Guidelines must be overlaid on the broader, and still developing industry standards, government statutory provisions and definitions for protecting and respecting privacy preferences. These industry standards include disclosure of what information is being collected and its intended uses, and the opportunity for the consumer to withhold consent for its collection for marketing purposes. Thus, in the case of Websites directed to children or children's portions of general audience sites that collect personal information from children, reasonable efforts, taking into consideration available technology, should be made to establish that notice is offered to, and choice exercised by a parent or guardian.

The availability of hyperlinks between sites can allow a child to move seamlessly from one to another. However there is no way to predict where the use of successive links on successive pages will lead. Therefore, operators of Websites for children or children's portions of general audience sites should not knowingly link to pages of other sites that do not comply with CARU's Guidelines.

In keeping with CARU's Principle regarding respecting and fostering the parents' role in providing guidance for their children, advertisers who communicate with children through email should remind and encourage parents to check and monitor their children's use of email and other online activities regularly.

To respect the privacy of parents, information collected and used for the sole purpose of obtaining verifiable parental consent or providing notice should not be maintained in retrievable form by the site if parental consent is not obtained after a reasonable time.

The following guidelines apply to online activities which are intentionally targeted to children under 13, or where the Website knows the visitor is a child. In Websites where there is a reasonable expectation that a significant number of children will be visiting, age-screening mechanisms should be employed to determine whether verifiable parental consent or notice and opt-out is necessitated per the Data Collection section of the Guidelines. These mechanisms should be used in conjunction with technology to help prevent an underage child from going back and changing his age to circumvent the age- screening. Care should be taken so that screening questions are asked in a neutral manner so as not to encourage children to provide inaccurate information to avoid obtaining parental permission.

For purposes of this section, these activities include making a sale or collecting data, and do not include the use of "spokescharacters" or branded environments for informational or entertainment purposes, which are addressed in the "Endorsement" and "Disclosure" sections of the Guidelines.

Making a Sale

Advertisers who transact sales with children online should make reasonable efforts in light of all available technologies to provide the person responsible for the costs of the transaction with the means to exercise control over the transaction. If there is no reasonable means provided to avoid unauthorized purchases of goods and services by children, the advertiser should enable the person responsible to cancel the order and receive full credit without incurring any charges. Advertisers should keep in mind that under existing state laws, parents may not be obligated to fulfill sales contracts entered into by their young children.

1. Children should always be told when they are being targeted for a sale.
2. If a site offers the opportunity to order or purchase any product or service, either through the use of a "click here to order" button or other on-screen means, the ordering instructions must clearly and prominently state that a child must have a parent's permission to order.
3. In the case of an online means of ordering, there should be a clear mechanism after the order is placed allowing the child or parent to cancel the order.

Data Collection

The ability to gather information, for marketing purposes, to tailor a site to a specific interest, etc., is part of the appeal of the interactive media to both the advertiser and the user. Young children however, may not understand the nature of the information being sought, nor its intended uses. The solicitation of personally identifiable information from children (e.g., full names, addresses, email addresses, phone numbers) triggers special privacy and security concerns.

Therefore, in collecting information from children under 13 years of age, advertisers should adhere to the following principles:

1. In all cases, the information collection or tracking practices and information uses must be clearly disclosed, along with the means of correcting or removing the information. The disclosure notice should be prominent and readily accessible before any information is collected. For instance, in the case of passive tracking, the notice should be on the page where the child enters the site. A heading such as "Privacy", "Our Privacy Policy", or similar designation which allows an adult to click on to obtain additional information on the site's information collection and tracking practices and information uses is acceptable.

2. When personal information (such as email addresses or screen names associated with other personal information) will be publicly posted so as to enable others to communicate directly with the child online, or when the child will be able otherwise to communicate directly with others, the company must obtain prior verifiable parental consent.

3. When personal information will be shared or distributed to third parties, except for parties that are agents or affiliates of the company or provide support for the internal operation of the Website and that agree not to disclose or use the information for any other purpose, the company must obtain prior verifiable parental consent.

4. When personal information is obtained for a company's internal use, and there is no disclosure, parental consent may be obtained through the use of email coupled with some additional steps to provide assurance that the person providing the consent is the parent.

5. When online contact information is collected and retained to respond directly more than once to a child's specific request (such as an email newsletter or contest) and will not be used for any other purpose, the company must directly notify the parent of the nature and intended uses of the information collected, and permit access to the information sufficient to permit a parent to remove or correct the information.

In furtherance of the above principles, advertisers should adhere to the following guidelines:

1. The advertiser should disclose, in language easily understood by a child, why the information is being requested (e.g., "We'll use your name and email to enter you in this contest and also add it to our mailing list") and whether the information is intended to be shared, sold or distributed outside of the collecting advertiser company.

2. If information is collected from children through passive means (e.g., navigational tracking tools, browser files, etc.) this should be disclosed along with what information is being collected.
3. Advertisers should encourage the child to use an alias (e.g., "Bookworm", "Skater", etc.), first name, nickname, initials, or other alternative to full names or screen names which correspond with an email address for any activities which will involve public posting.
4. The operator should not require a child to disclose more personal information than is reasonably necessary to participate in the online activity (e.g., play a game, enter a contest, etc.).
5. The interactivity of the medium offers the opportunity to communicate with children through electronic mail. While this is part of the appeal of the medium, it creates the potential for a child to receive unmanageable amounts of unsolicited email. If an advertiser communicates with a child by email, there should be an opportunity with each mailing for the child or parent to choose by return email to discontinue receiving mailings.

Guidelines for the Advertising of 900/976 Teleprograms to Children

These guidelines, promulgated in 1989, have been superseded by a prohibition by the Federal Trade Commission that pay-per-call services cannot be directed to children under 12, unless the service is a "bona fide educational service." Likewise, ads for 900-number services cannot be directed to children under 12, unless the service is a bona fide educational service per section 308.3 (d)(I) of the Rule Pursuant to the Telephone Disclosure and Dispute Resolution Act of 1992.

APPENDIX C.
GROCERY MANUFACTURERS OF
AMERICA PROPOSAL ON CARU GUIDES

Written Submission of Manly Molpus
President and CEO, Grocery Manufacturers Association
On Behalf of
Campbell Soup Company; General Mills, Inc.; The Hershey Company;
Kellogg Company; Kraft Foods Inc.; Nestlé USA; PepsiCo, Inc.; Sara Lee
Corporation; Unilever United States, Inc.
Federal Trade Commission and Department of Health and Human Services
Public Workshop on Marketing, Self Regulation and Childhood Obesity
July 15, 2005

Proposals to Strengthen Advertising Self-Regulation and to Encourage Public-Private Initiatives Promoting Healthy Lifestyles

We would like to thank Secretary Leavitt and FTC Chairman Majoras for their leadership in building understanding around the role of marketing in fostering healthy children's lifestyles. We particularly appreciate this opportunity for the food and beverage industry to participate in the FTC-HHS workshop on July 14-15.

As companies in the food and beverage industry who are also supporters of CARU, we recognize that we have a unique opportunity to help make a spectrum of food choices available to everyone, especially to children, and to use our marketing resources to promote both healthy eating and healthy activity choices. In support of that, we also understand that meaningful, robust self-regulation of children's marketing is in everyone's interest.

We believe the self-regulatory system managed by the National Advertising Review Council and implemented through the National Advertising Division ("NAD") and the Children's Advertising Review Unit ("CARU") has worked well over the years and ensures that advertising meets the highest standards of truth and accuracy. We believe self-regulation can be an even more effective tool and that CARU, in particular, can play a major role in that effort.

In that spirit, we have offered our support to the NAD and CARU for strengthening their efforts in several important respects. In suggesting these improvements, we strongly believe that CARU can continue to be the standard for strong, effective, and credible self- regulation of advertising that American consumers can count on. We will re-commit ourselves to that goal and pledge our companies to providing the financial support that is required.

1. *Build CAR U's resources and enforcement capacity.* We believe that CARU staff and resources must be substantially increased in order to effectively implement several of the recommendations suggested here. In addition to ensuring adequate enforcement capacity, expanded staff will allow CARU to continuously improve its effectiveness, and to ensure improved consumer access as described below.

2. *Improve direct consumer access.* We believe consumers, especially parents, should have immediate and direct access to CARU for purposes of expressing concerns about specific advertisements and about children's advertising in general. That could be accomplished by establishing a toll-free consumer response line and website, publicizing the existence of both, and responding to consumers directly regarding complaints and comments.

3. *Improve transparency.* We believe a summary of CARU's regulatory activities should be available to the public on the CARU website and should include a review of complaints filed, against whom, and on what general topic, in addition to final resolutions of those complaints. While such information is provided in written reports to subscribers and is public information, we believe the website ought to provide easy access to an overview of the scope of CARU's regulatory activities.

4. *Broaden involvement and advice to CARU on matters of children's health.* We support augmenting CARU's external advisory boards to provide more expertise on matters related to health, wellness and nutrition and including parents, educators, nutritionists, fitness experts, behavioral experts, and experts on FTC and FDA policy. The expanded advisory board could:
   - Provide expert guidance to the CARU staff during the advertising monitoring and review process.
   - Advise the National Advertising Review Council on suggested improvements to the existing guidelines.
   - Work with advertisers to develop approaches that encourage constructive and consistent healthy lifestyle messages.

5. *Strengthen voluntary pre-dissemination review of ads.* We support strengthening the existing mechanism for pre-review of advertising with

the goal of preventing advertising that is not consistent with CARU's guidelines from reaching the marketplace. We envision this as a voluntary mechanism that could be strengthened through the participation by members of an expanded staff and advisory board.

6. *Ensure CAR U's guidelines address certain marketing practices as follows*:

   - Expand CARU's guidelines to address advertising contained in commercial computer games, video games and interactive websites.
   - Prohibit paid product placement on children's programming.
   - Appropriate use of third-party licensed characters in advertising.

7. *Build a closer working relationship with FTC and HHS.* We believe robust self- regulation requires effective support from both industry and government. To that end, we would encourage the FTC to look for ways to strengthen its relationship with CARU.

In addition, we believe that government can play a role in helping support private sector initiatives to promote healthy lifestyles. In that regard, we have two recommendations:

1. *Develop an HHS award program that recognizes companies for promoting healthy lifestyles.* We believe that healthy lifestyles originate with healthy environments and individual choices. The private sector, across a wide range of industries, can make a significant contribution by helping to provide consumers with the knowledge, motivation and options to make healthy choices and build healthy habits. An HHS-sponsored program that defines and recognizes meaningful contributions in areas such as employee health and wellness, community activities, consumer communications, product development and public-private partnerships could have a significant impact in mobilizing private sector actions.

2. *Maintain federal funding for healthy lifestyle communication programs, like the HHS/Ad Council "Small Steps" campaign and the CDC's VERB program or successor* campaign. By supporting the development of comprehensive communication programs, among a wide constituency, the government is not only building awareness, particularly among children, but is substantially contributing to the knowledge base around successful behavioral interventions.

Once we've received feedback on our suggestions for strengthening self-regulation from FTC, HHS and other stakeholders at the Workshop, we propose that a task force be assembled to move these ideas swiftly forward, with a fixed deadline for finalizing an implementation plan for the agreed-upon improvements.

Thank you for your efforts to further understanding and promote constructive solutions. We look forward to your reactions and would welcome further discussions.

APPENDIX D.
NATIONAL ADVERTISING REVIEW COUNCIL RESPONSE TO GMA PROPOSAL

September 15, 2005

Mr. Donald S. Clark
Federal Trade Commission
Office of the Secretary
Room 159-H (Annex H)
600 Pennsylvania Avenue,
NW Washington, DC 20580

Mr. C. Manly Molpus
President and Chief Executive Officer
Grocery Manufacturers Association
2401 Pennsylvania Avenue, NW, 2nd Floor
Washington, DC 20037

RE: Food Marketing to Kids Workshop - Comment, Project No. P034519

Dear Messrs. Clark and Molpus:

The National Advertising Review Council (NARC) would like to offer further comment regarding the Federal Trade Commission (FTC) and Health and Human Services (HMS) Workshop on Marketing, Self-Regulation and Childhood Obesity. This letter will provide an update on certain works in progress to reinforce and improve the children's advertising review program, administered by the Children's Advertising Review Unit (CARU) of the Council of Better

Business Bureaus (CBBB). In doing so, it will address the positive suggestions presented by the Grocery Manufacturers Association (GMA) during the Workshop on behalf of a number of its member companies, and made part of the Workshop record.

Policies for CARU are set by NARC, relying on the practical experience of industry advertising experts and the self-regulatory experience of the CBBB. We are pleased to have been offered the opportunity to participate in the Workshop and to be able to present CARUs record of effectiveness in maintaining a robust, independent and transparent system of self-regulation that has been in place for more than 30 years. We applaud the industry for its compliance rate of more than 95 percent with CARU decisions. We welcome the continued and increased support to which the food industry is committed.

CARU's mandate is clear - to monitor and evaluate advertising messages to children, in all media, for compliance with its *Self-Regulatory Guidelines for Children's Advertising* (the *Guidelines),* many of which impose limitations far beyond those imposed by any law or regulation. CARU was created to ensure that advertising directed to children is truthful, accurate, and appropriate for its intended audience. It is important to recognize that CARU was not established to be the arbiter of which products should or should not be manufactured, sold, or marketed to children, or to tell parents or children which products they should or shouldn't buy.

Within CARU's mandate, summarized below are some key initiatives being undertaken by CARU, with the support of NARC, to address issues raised at the Workshop.

Improve Direct Consumer Access

CARU has recently established a complaint form on its Website that facilitates receipt of consumer complaints and other contacts with CARU regarding traditional or online media. In addition to the easily accessed complaint form, CARU is at or near the top of the list when one conducts an Internet search on Google, Yahoo! or AltaVista for "children's advertising" or "complain about advertising to children." To make CARU even more broadly visible and accessible to consumers, the CBBB has created a link to the "File a Complaint" pages of the more than 100 Better Business Bureaus as well as BBBOnLine, which may be accessed through the BBB's main Website, *www.bbb.org.* The Websites which link to the complaint system attract over 20 million visitors annually. The complaint pages themselves generate over 200,000 visits.

In addition to the visibility afforded through the BBB's Website, the other three NARC partners -the Association of National Advertisers (ANA), the American Association of Advertising Agencies (AAAA) and the American Advertising Federation (AAF) - have agreed to provide links to CARU's Website. The CARU Website already has links from industry associations including the GMA, the Toy Industry Association (TIA) and the American Bar Association (ABA). SEARCH: The National Consortium for Justice Information and Statistics, an organization formed by the 50 states' governors to provide quality information on new technology to statewide law enforcement agencies, links to CARU. Additionally, there are links to CARU from law schools and universities in several states and in Canada. We will encourage additional industry, educational and public-interest organization links.

Our goal is to ensure an accessible, user-friendly CARU complaint process that will constantly expand and allow CARU to gather as much relevant information as possible about the claims, time, place, and medium involved in an advertisement. This online complaint procedure (in addition to postal mail and telephone services) is predicated on successful experiences acquired through the BBB system as well as the U.K. and Canadian self-regulatory systems. After full implementation, we will evaluate the effectiveness of the system and the need to consider (or expand to include) other potential systems including, if appropriate, a toll-free number.

Improve Transparency

Transparency is a key attribute for an effective self-regulatory system. Accordingly, CARU and the National Advertising Division (NAD) of the CBBB publish their decisions. National self- regulation is not a confidential mediation or arbitration procedure. CARU's press releases describing its case decisions have always been made available free to all upon request and, since its Website was launched, through its Website. The press releases are transmitted immediately to a press distribution list, which is provided access to the entire case decision as well. Earlier this year, NARC created and filled the position of director of communications to help heighten CARU's public profile.

For several years, CARU and NAD have expanded access to their work through a subscription system that provides an online searchable and printable database of CARU and NAD case decisions. The archive includes all cases opened by CARU and NAD and is searchable by advertiser, brand, product category, chronologically and by date range.

Although members of the general public have been able to obtain individual case decisions free upon request, we recognize that we may be able to ease access, particularly for non-profit organizations that may have a need for decisions on more than a case-by-case basis. Accordingly, NARC is in the process of developing a system by which the public, as well as bona fide public-interest and educational institutions, can more easily access the existing archive of cases through a free subscription. Additionally, once developed, NARC will announce the availability of these archives and will also contact educational, consumer, and parent community groups who might have an interest in these archives.

Broadened Involvement and Advice to CARU on Matters of Children's Health

At the time CARU was established, it was widely understood that children are not just "little adults" and that their cognitive abilities are more limited than those of older children or adults.

It was with this in mind that CBBB established CARU and NARC brought it under the umbrella of the existing, successful advertising self-regulation program it sponsored. CARU was established with an advisory board of experts in child development, to look beyond truth and accuracy in ensuring that advertising messages directed to children were clear and understandable to their intended audience.

CARU recognizes that professional expertise from individuals knowledgeable in the areas of education, communication, child mental health and nutrition is crucial. Accordingly, CARU consults with its Academic Advisory Board, composed of leading experts in these fields. These experts assist CARU in the review and application of the *Guidelines.* When a particular ad raises questions about children's perception or cognitive ability to comprehend the message, for example, CARU staff seeks the expert advice of the Academic Advisory Board before opening an inquiry. In the past year, CARU has expanded the board, adding two nutritionists to the already-included experts in child psychiatry, developmental psychology and childhood communications.

With NARC's encouragement and CBBB's support, CARU will continue to expand this group to provide broader input and access to experts who will help guide its decisions. Further, NARC has approved policy changes that will increase the transparency of the program by making any expert opinion relied upon by CARU available to the advertiser and complainants in that case.

NARC is also asking CARU to broaden and enhance its industry support advisory group so that it is inclusive to represent all CARU Supporters. Along with the academic and other experts, this group will better provide valuable insight on children's advertising issues and trends pertinent to the self-regulation program.

It is not the goal or focus of self regulation to provide the industry with specific programs or approaches addressing health issues. In fact, the Advertising Council, supported and funded in part by the trade association members of NARC, has developed programs to help advertisers develop approaches that encourage constructive and consistent healthy lifestyle messages and, when appropriate, we offer the Ad Council NARC's support.

Strengthen Voluntary Pre-Dissemination Review of Ads

Pre-screening of all forms of advertising has long been available as a benefit to CARU Supporters. We agree that this process may help prevent advertising inconsistent with CARU *Guidelines* from reaching the marketplace, but the use of this service is, and will remain, voluntary. NARC has, however, asked CARU to expand this opportunity to pre-screen and, accordingly, CARU will make its voluntary pre-screening process available to non-Supporters at a reasonable fee.

We appreciate and welcome the GMA and its members encouraging greater awareness of this voluntary pre-screening opportunity for both CARU Supporters and non-Supporters.

Ensure CAR U's Guidelines Address Certain Marketing Practices

- *Expand CAR U's Guidelines to address advertising contained in commercial computer games, video games and interactive Websites*

CARU's *Guidelines,* as currently applied, do address advertising to children on interactive Websites and CARU routinely reviews these Websites.

Further, CARU has appointed a task force to explore the extent to which new forms of online offerings are included within the self-regulation system's definition of "national advertising," or if not, whether they should be. The task force has been asked to report back to CARU in mid-September. Upon receipt of that report, CARU will prepare a recommendation to the NARC Board for final approval and possible revision of the *Guidelines.*

CARU is also exploring efficient ways to monitor advertising addressed to children on computer and video games.

- *Prohibit paid product placement on children's programmin•*

CARU is unaware of any current paid product placement in children's television programming, as defined by CARU. However, in order to ensure that its approach to this issue is the appropriate one, NARC has asked CARU to form a task force to determine whether children's programming contains product placement, and if so, whether disclosures or any other approach would be meaningful to children.

- *Appropriate use of third-party licensed characters in advertising*

CARU currently applies its *Guidelines* to all advertising directed to children, including advertising utilizing licensed characters. The *Guidelines* specifically prohibit "host selling" situations. Host selling occurs when a live or animated personality is used to sell products or services in, or adjacent to, programs primarily directed to children in which the same personality or character appears.

Because broader issues suggested by the GMA letter would impact a number of industry segments and constituents whose input is valuable and necessary for further NARC consideration, we will initiate discussion to gather that input.

- *Build a Closer Relationship With the FTC and HHS*

NARC and CARU have long enjoyed a strong relationship with FTC, as have NAD and the Electronic Retailing Self-Regulation Program (ERSP). NARC agrees that these relationships should be enhanced and extended to HHS. To that end, in addition to our regular ongoing contacts, we would like to renew a practice of the self-regulation system that hasn't been used in recent years: an annual formal NARC briefing to the FTC on current issues, cases and trends.

This briefing will be provided by the NARC partners to all FTC commissioners, and NARC will work to arrange a similar relationship with HHS.

We look forward to working with the GMA and the rest of the children's advertising industry to enhance the current process, public awareness and public confidence in the self-regulatory system.

Cordially,

James R. Guthrie
President and CEO
National Advertising Review Council
cc: NARC Board
     CARU Supporters

ENDNOTES

1. The Federal Advisory Committee Act ("FACA"), 5 U.S.C. App. Sect. 3(2), does not apply to the workshop for a number of reasons. First, the workshop was convened for the purpose of assisting industry in developing self-regulatory guidelines, not for the purpose of obtaining advice or recommendations for the agencies. 41 C.F.R. Sect. 102-3.25; *see Sofamor Danek Group, Inc. v. Gaus*, 61 F. 3d 929 (D.C. Cir. 1995), *cert. denied* 516 U.S. 1112 (1996). Second, participation in the discussions at the workshop was open to the public via a public mike, providing a chance for any individual to voice opinions and share information, and thus did not incorporate the kind of management or control applicable to advisory committees. 41 C.F.R. Sect. 102-3 App. A to Subpart A, Sect. II. Third, it was a meeting for the purpose of exchanging facts or information, 41 C.F.R. Sect. 102-3.40(f). Finally, even if, to some extent, advice for the agencies may have been sought from or provided by attendees, it was sought or provided on an individual basis and not from the group as a whole. 41 C.F.R. Sect. 102-3.40(e).

2. For children, the terms "overweight" and "obesity" are used interchangeably and are defined as a BMI at or above the 95th percentile for gender and age (BMI-for-age) in children. *See* Centers for Disease Control and Prevention, "BMI - Body Mass Index: BMI for Children and Teens," http://www.cdc.gov/nccdphp/dnpa/bmi/bmi-for-age.htm. For adults, a BMI of 25-29 denotes someone who is overweight and a BMI of 30 or more denotes obesity.

    Throughout this chapter citations to "Tr. I" and "Tr. II" refer to the transcript of the workshop. "Tr. I" citations refer to the transcript of the July 14 proceedings, and "Tr. II" to the July 15 proceedings. Speakers are identified by last name. The full transcript is available at http://www.ftc.gov/bcp/workshops/foodmarketingtokids/transcript_050714.pdf and 050715.pdf.

3. National Center for Health Statistics, "Prevalence of Overweight Among Children and Adolescents: United States, 1999-2002," http://www.cdc.gov/nchs/products/pubs/pubd/hestats/ overwght99.htm (last visited Mar. 10, 2006); Carmona, Tr. II at 7-8 ("[w]e can track this trend over the last several decades").

4. Richard P. Troiano and Katherine M. Flegal, "Overweight Children and Adolescents: Description, Epidemiology, and Demographics," 101 Pediatrics 497-504 (1998).

5. The 1999-2000 National Health and Nutrition Examination Survey ("NHANES") found that African American and Mexican American adolescents ages 12-19 were more likely to be overweight, at 21 percent and 23 percent respectively, than non-Hispanic white adolescents (14 percent). *See* National Center for Health Statistics, "Obesity Still a Major Problem, New Data Show," http://www.cdc.gov/nchs/pressroom/04facts/obesity.htm. In children 6-11 years old, 22 percent of Mexican American children were overweight, whereas 20 percent of African American children and 14 percent of non-Hispanic white children were overweight. *Id.*

6. Carmona, Tr. II at 8 ("Childhood obesity is an epidemic ... and is a significant problem.").

7. Dietz, Tr. I at 48.

8. According to a prospective study conducted in Bogalusa, Louisiana, researchers found that half of adults with a BMI that is greater than 40 (roughly 100 pounds overweight or more), were likely to have been overweight during childhood. *Id.* at 49-50.

9. Centers for Disease Control and Prevention, "Physical Activity and Good Nutrition: Essential Elements to Prevent Chronic Diseases and Obesity," http://www.cdc.gov/nccdphp/aag/aag_dnpa.htm; Dietz, Tr. I at 43-46.

10. Harbour, Tr. I at 139 ("education can play a key part in helping parents and children take responsibility for smart eating choices."); Carmona, Tr. II at 14-15 (consumer education is needed to improve health literacy among Americans).

11. Crawford, Tr. I at 19; Carmona, Tr. II at 17 (the 2005 Dietary Guidelines will help improve health literacy among Americans).

12. *See* USDA website at http://teamnutrition.usda.gov/kids-pyramid.html.

13. Crawford, Tr. I at 20; *see* http://wecan.nhlbi.nih.gov.

14. *See* http://www.cdc.gov/youthcampaign/.

15. Crawford, Tr. I at 23.

16. *See* http://www.healthierus.gov/steps/.

[17.] Crawford, Tr. I at 20-22. Among other things, the FDA is considering whether calorie information should be made more prominent on the food label, whether serving sizes for some foods need to be updated, and whether multiple serving packages that could reasonably be consumed as a single serving should have calories listed on the label for both a single serving and the entire package, or for just the entire package. *See* 70 Fed. Reg. 17,008 (April 4, 2005).

[18.] The Keystone Center for Science and Public Policy is an organization that provides independent facilitator and mediation services to build consensus among public, private, and civic sectors in areas of environmental, health, and energy policy.

[19.] Crawford, Tr. I at 24-25.

[20.] *Id.*

[21.] Although the majority of those cases have involved weight loss products marketed for adults, a few have challenged allegedly deceptive claims for products promoted as weight loss aids for children. *See, e.g., FTC v. The Fountain of Youth Group, LLC,* Civil Action No. 3:04-CV-47-J 99HTS (M.D. Fla. Feb. 10, 2004) (stipulated final order) (challenged weight loss claims included advertising for "Skinny Pill for Kids").

[22.] "Deception in Weight-Loss Advertising Workshop: Seizing Opportunities and Building Partnerships to Stop Weight Loss Fraud: A Federal Trade Commission Staff Report," at ii (Dec. 2003), *available at* http://www.ftc.gov/os/2003/12/031209weightlossrpt.pdf.

[23.] "2004 Weight-Loss Advertising Survey: Staff Report: Federal Trade Commission," (Apr. 2005), *available at* http://www.ftc.gov/os/2005/04/050411weightlosssurvey04.pdf.

[24.] Decision to Terminate Rulemaking, *In the Matter of Children's Advertising,* 46 Fed. Reg. 48,710 (1981); *see also* Howard Beales, III, "Advertising to Kids and the FTC," 12 Geo. Mason Law Rev. 873 (2004).

[25.] *See, e.g., Lorillard Tobacco Co. v. Reilly,* 533 U.S. 525, 534-36 (2001) (striking down state restrictions on outdoor placement of tobacco advertising), *see also* Majoras, Tr. I at 9-10.

[26.] Majoras, Tr. I at 9-10.

[27.] The workshop was also a response to a recommendation by the Institute of Medicine of the National Academy of Sciences ("IOM"). In 2004, the IOM's Committee on Prevention of Obesity in Children and Youth issued a report with many recommendations for industry, government, school, and parental action to combat childhood obesity. Institute of Medicine, *Preventing Childhood Obesity: Health in the Balance,* The National Academies Press (2005) (hereinafter "IOM Childhood Obesity Report"). The IOM recommended that HHS convene a public conference to assist in the development of industry self-regulatory guidelines for marketing and advertising to children. The IOM also recommended that the FTC monitor compliance with the guidelines.

[28.] Majoras, Tr. I at 10; *see also* Harbour, Tr. I at 142 ("I also encourage food marketers and the media to consider adopting a set of best practices.").

[29.] Throughout this report the terms "food industry" and "food companies" refer collectively to all parties engaged in the marketing of foods and beverages and include the restaurant industry.

[30.] Majoras, Tr. I at 12-14.

[31.] This report mentions specific companies and their products. These references do not constitute an endorsement by FTC or HHS of these companies or their products.

[32.] *Id.*

[33.] The report attempts to illustrate the range of techniques used to market foods to children and the variety of industry initiatives to address childhood obesity concerns. Various sections highlight examples of the actions of specific members of the food and media industries. Most of the examples are drawn from those companies who participated in the workshop or filed comments. The report is not necessarily representative of the companies that did not participate, nor does it provide a comprehensive account of industry conduct.

[34.] A recently completed evidentiary review and analysis of food marketing and children's diets and health, by the Institute of Medicine's Committee on Food Marketing and the Diets of Children and Youth, noted significant gaps in the research. In particular, the IOM Committee's report notes that much of the relevant marketing research and data are proprietary and that peer- reviewed literature on the role of food marketing in the diets of children is largely limited to television advertising and has not explored other marketing venues and techniques. Institute of Medicine, *Food Marketing to Children and Youth: Threat or Opportunity?*, The National Academies Press (2005) (hereinafter "IOM Food Marketing Report"), *available at* http://www.nap.edu/ catalog/11514.html. Congress recently directed the FTC to conduct a food marketing study examining and attempting to quantify the full range of food marketing activities and expenditures directed at children and adolescents, including television, radio, print and Internet advertising, packaging, promotional events, in-store marketing, and product placement. Conference Report (H.R. Rep. No. 109-272 (2005)) for Pub. L. No. 109-108 (incorporating by reference language from the Senate Report (S. Rep. No. 109-88 (2005)).

35. IOM Childhood Obesity Report at 198-99. IOM estimates that, in 2002, the food industry spent about $1 billion to advertise foods in television and print media to children, out of a total $10 to $12 billion spent on food marketing to children.

36. The IOM Food Marketing Report describes and attempts to quantify the variety of marketing techniques and venues used by food companies to reach children. IOM Food Marketing Report, Chapter 4.

37. Campaign for a Commercial-Free Childhood ("CCFC") Comment at 3. All public comments submitted in connection with the workshop are available at http://www.ftc.gov/os/comments/FoodMarketingtoKids/index.htm.

38. Spending by children aged 4 to 12 is estimated to exceed $50 billion annually, while spending by teenagers is estimated at over $150 billion annually. *See* Market Research.com, *Kids and Money* (July 13, 2001), *available at* http://www.marketresearch.com.

39. IOM Childhood Obesity Report at 200, *citing* H. Stipp, "New Ways to Reach Children," 14 *Amer. Demog.* 50 (1993); *see also* IOM Food Marketing Report at 1-4 (citing to more recent research estimating that children and youth collectively spend more than $200 billion annually).

40. IOM Childhood Obesity Report at 178. The IOM Food Marketing Report found a similar emphasis on food purchases, estimating that of the various spending categories, one-third of children's direct purchases are for sweets, snacks, and beverages, followed by toys and apparel. IOM Food Marketing Report at 1-4.

41. *Id.* at 198-99 (*citing* M. Nestle, Food Politics: How the Food Industry Influences Nutrition and Health (2003); K. Brownell, Food Fight: The Inside Story of the Food Industry, America's Obesity Crisis and What We Can Do About It (2004)).

42. The IOM Food Marketing Report notes that total marketing investments by the food industry have not been clearly identified, but estimates that "only approximately 20% of all food and beverage marketing in 2004 was devoted to advertising on television, radio, print, billboards or the Internet," and suggests that, while television remains an important vehicle, a shift is occurring toward other forms of marketing, such as product placement, character licensing, special events, in-school activities, and advergames. IOM Food Marketing Report, at ES-3.

43. *See* FTC Staff Report, *Slotting Allowances in the Retail Grocery Industry: Selected Case Studies of Slotting Allowances in Five Product Categories* (2003); *see also* Childs, Tr. I at 89.

44. *See* http://www.mcdonalds.com/usa/ronald/happy.html (as visited Aug. 2, 2005).

45. *See* http://www.keebler.com/promotions/magicbythemillion/rules.shtml (as visited Aug. 2, 2005).

46. *See Marketing Practices* in the Grocery Industry at 10 (Feb. 2001), *available at* http://www.ftc.gov/os/2001/02/slottingallowancesreport-final.pdf. For another example of a McDonald's toy tie-in, see Rideout Presentation.

47. *See* CCFC Comment at 5.

48. *See* CIFC Comment (June 7, 2005) at 9 (when brands appear on children's products, the children themselves become advertisements for the product). According to James McNeal, a professor of marketing at Texas A&M University who specializes in marketing to children, "licensed fads have a snowball effect. As they buy and display licensed products, the children are becoming salespeople, of sorts, for the licensed products." Consumers Union, "Selling America's Kids: Commercial Pressures on Kids of the 90's" (1998), *available at* www.consumersunion.ort/other/sellingkids/license.htm.

49. *See* http://1 64.109.46.215/1 00/innovations/kraftmac.html

50. *See* Stephanie Thompson, "General Mills Adds Disney Characters to Fruit Snacks Line," *Advertising Age* (May 8, 2000), at 22.

51. *Id.*

52. FCC regulations requiring buffers between programming and commercial content effectively prohibit product placement on children's television programming, but children see such placements when watching family programming such as *American Idol. See* Children's Television Act of 1990, 47 U.S.C. § 303a, and implementing regulation, 47 C.F.R. § 76.225.

53. The IOM cited an estimate that food companies spent $3 billion in 2002 on packaging designed to appeal to children. IOM Childhood Obesity Report at 199, *citing* McNeal.

54. Harkin, Tr. I at 39; Smalls, Tr. I at 282-83.

55. Packaging size, such as smaller portion sizes or resealable packages, also can also have an impact on the level of consumption. *See* IOM Childhood Obesity Report at 182, 184.

56. *See* Center for Science and the Public Interest, *Pestering Parents: How Food Companies Market Obesity to Children* at 23-24 (Nov. 10, 2003), at 23-24, *available at* http://www.cspinet.org/new/200311101.html (hereinafter "*Pestering Parents*").

57. The IOM has cited an estimate that food companies spent $2 billion in 2002 on public relations efforts. IOM Childhood Obesity Report at 199, *citing* McNeal.

58. *See* General Accounting Office (as of 2004, the "Government Accountability Office"), *Commercial Activities in Schools* at 28-31 (Sept. 2000).

59. *See Pestering Parents* at 31-32.

60. The IOM has cited an estimate that food companies spent $1 billion on traditional advertising. IOM Childhood Obesity Report at 199, *citing* McNeal.

61. Advertising Age, *Special Report: 1,000 Leading National Advertisers* (Jun. 27, 2005), at S 14.

62. The IOM's recent report on food marketing reviewed the available studies on children's exposure to advertising on television. The findings of these studies vary considerably, depending on when they were done, the method and data used to estimate exposure, and whether the study adjusts for the increased use of 15-second ads over time. *See* IOM Food Marketing Report at 4-41 - 4-43.

63. The FTC staff relied on Nielsen data for one week in each of November 2003, February, May and July 2004. The data cover ads in seven broadcast networks, 50 national ad-supported cable networks, nationally syndicated programming, and ads that originate locally.

64. *See* John D. Abel, *The Child Audience for Network Television Programming and Advertising,* (Nov. 1978) (a study of national TV advertising to children); J. Howard Beales, III, *An Analysis of Exposure to Non-Network Television Advertising,* (Nov. 1978) (a study of local advertising exposure); and Richard P. Adler *et al., Research on the Effects of Television Advertising on Children,* National Science Foundation (GPO, Washington, D.C. 1977) (a review of children's TV viewing patterns). Both the 1977 and 2004 ad data are from sweeps months so the ad composition may differ from that in other months.

65. Children's shows are those in which children make up at least 50 percent of the audience; family shows are those in which children make up at least 20 percent of the audience.

66. The IOM's recent report also reviewed available studies on food advertising to children, especially in children's television programming. The largest studies reviewed by IOM suggest that food advertising was 64 percent of ads in children's programming in the 1970s, 52 percent in the 1 980s, and 46 percent in the early 1 990s. *See* IOM Food Marketing Report at 4-44.

67. CSS/GES Comment at 6.

68. Screenshots of examples can be found at http://www.ftc.gov/bcp/ workshops/foodmarketingtokids/presentations/vrideout.pdf. For additional examples of web- based food advertising, *see Pestering Parents* at 20-21.

69. Story and French Comment at 9; *see also* Moore, Tr. I at 12 1-22.

70. Advertising Age, Special Report, at S-14.

71. McIntyre, Tr. I at 102-03; Moore, Tr. I at 121.

72. Majoras, Tr. I at 8-9; Carmona, Tr. II at 8-10. This view is consistent with that of other researchers and advocates. *See, e.g.*, IOM Report at 181-92, 198-204; Promotion Marketing Association, Inc., Comment at 5; Sandy Szwarc, Comment at 2. *See also* Todd Zywicki, Debra Holt & Maureen Ohlhausen, "Obesity and Advertising Policy," 12 Geo. Mason L. Rev. 979 (2004).

73. Comment of the Association of National Advertisers ("ANA"), June 7, 2005 at 4; Comment of the Grocery Manufacturers Association ("GMA"), July 14, 2005 at 10; Byrd-Bredbenner, Tr. I at 234-5.

74. Previous research has documented ways in which marketing can have positive health benefits. In the 1 980s, food advertising on the link between fiber and cancer risk led to increased consumer demand for high fiber cereals and increased the supply of products with higher fiber. *See* Pauline Ippolito & Alan Mathios, *Health Claims in Advertising and Labeling: A Study of the Cereal Market*, FTC Bureau of Economic Staff Report (1989).

75. Goldin, Tr. I at 167; Jaffe, Tr. II at 115.

76. A 2005 survey by the GMA showed that 86% of the 42 food and beverage companies responding to the survey were introducing new products or reformulating products and sizes, with another 12% planning to do so. Since 2002, those 42 companies had introduced 4,500 new or reformulated products and sizes. GMA Health & Wellness Initiative Survey (July 2005), *appended to* GMA Comment, at 4-6.

77. *See, e.g.,* Berlind, Tr. I at 212; Leach, Tr. I at 213 and Tr. II at 138.

78. *See, e.g.,* Goldin, Tr. I at 19 1-92.

79. General Mills Comment at 2; Byrd-Bredbenner, Tr. I at 237; Leach, Tr. I at 241.

80. Berlind, Tr. I at 239.

81. Harris, Tr. I at 2 19, 242-43.

82. Rodgers, Tr. I at 151.

83. Pepsi Comment at 1; Kraft Presentation, Slide 4.

84. Donahue, Tr. I at 159.

85. Kellogg Comment at 3.

86. GMA Health and Wellness Initiatives Survey (July 2005), at 5.

87. Donahue, Tr. I at 159.

88. Kellogg Comment at 4.

89. Berlind, Tr. I at 212; Leach, Tr. I at 214.

90. According to General Mills, this conversion means that all of its cereals are now either an excellent or good source of whole grain, as defined by the company. The purpose of the conversion to whole grain was purportedly to

improve heart health and help with weight management. General Mills Comment at 7-8.

[91.] Kraft Comment at 3.

[92.] Leach, Tr. I at 218, Pepsi Presentation at Slide 8.

[93.] In its 2003 report on food marketing to children, CSPI praised the fact that some companies are offering a few more nutritious choices for children but also asserted that little overall progress had been made. *Pestering Parents* at 51.

[94.] CIFC Comment (June 7, 2005) at 7.

[95.] The GMA survey found that more than half of the food and beverage companies it surveyed had made packaging changes specifically to create sizes more appropriate for children. GMA Health and Wellness Initiatives Survey (July 2005), *appended to* GMA Comment, at 7.

[96.] Powell, Tr. I at 148-9.

[97.] *Id.*

[98.] Leach, Tr. I at 215; Rodgers, Tr. I at 151; Kellogg Comment at 5; Berlind, Tr. I at 208.

[99.] Donahue, Tr. I at 159.

[100.] General Mills Comment at 3-4.

[101.] *See, e.g.,* Berlind, Tr. I at 241-2.

[102.] Powell, Tr. I at 149.

[103.] *See* http://www.dole.com/Products/Products_Detail.jsp?CatGroupID=5&ID= 42.

[104.] Harris, Tr. I at 221, 248;

[105.] Sutherland, Tr. I at 171; Leach, Tr. I at 216, 249.

[106.] Berlind, Tr. I at 212.

[107.] Reeves, Tr. I at 175; Byrd-Bredbenner, Tr. I at 236; Leach, Tr. I at 255; Acuff, Tr. I at 266.

[108.] Sutherland, Tr. I at 168-71,182-83 and 194; Acuff, Tr. I at 228.

[109.] Kraft Comment at 4; Berlind, Tr. I at 211.

[110.] Pepsi Presentation; Leach, Tr. I at 215.

[111.] Harris, Tr. I at 221.

[112.] General Mills Comment at 8-9; Powell, Tr. I at 148-49.

[113.] Berlind, Tr. I at 212.

[114.] Leach, Tr. I at 217.

[115.] *Id.* at 216; Harris, Tr. I at 221. Pepsi, for example, reported testing a stop light format that has been adopted in other countries. According to Pepsi, consumers hated the idea of a warning signal on products. They preferred being told what was healthier rather than being made to feel guilty about foods they already recognized had unhealthy attributes. Leach, Tr. I at 249.

[116.] Berlind, Tr. I at 246; Leach, Tr. I at 247.

[117.] CIFC Comment (June 7, 2005) at 13-14.

[118.] Berlind, Tr. I at 246; Leach, Tr. I at 246.

[119.] FDA food labeling regulations include definitions of a variety of terms that are permitted on food packaging to characterize the level of nutrients in a food, such as "good source," "low," and "reduced." To the extent these or similar terms are incorporated into company nutrition icons on product labels, they would need to be consistent with FDA labeling regulations.

[120.] *Id.*; McKinnon, Tr. I at 247.

[121.] Leach, Tr. I at 247.

[122.] Harris, Tr. I at 249.

[123.] Berlind, Tr. I at 250. One participant suggested that, in addition to providing signals on packaged food, there is also a need for clear cues in supermarkets and restaurants to help consumers make healthier choices. Byrd-Bredbenner, Tr. I at 252.

[124.] GMA Comment at 4.

[125.] Kellogg Comment at 4-5.

[126.] Leach, Tr. I at 215.

[127.] Kraft Comment at 4.

[128.] *See* Rhonda Rundle, *Read It and Weep? Big Mac Wrapper to Show Fat, Calories*, Wall Street Journal, Oct. 26, 2005 at B1. Foods sold in restaurants are not generally subject to the FDA labeling regulations that require disclosure of nutrition information on packaged food labeling.

[129.] Rodgers, Tr. I at 153.

[130.] Kraft Comment at 3.

[131.] Berlind, Tr. I at 211.

[132.] Leach, Tr. I at 218.

[133.] CCFC Comment at 3. As an example, CCFC points to Coca-Cola's sponsorship of *American Idol,* a program that consistently rated among the top ten shows viewed by children ages 2 to 11.

[134.] CIFC Comment at (June 7, 2005) 7-9 (June 7, 2005).

[135.] Produce for Better Health Foundation, "National Action Plan to Promote Health Through Increased Fruit and Vegetable Consumption" (2005) at 4, *available at* http://www.5aday.org/commcenter/actionplan/pbh_nap_book041905.pdf.

[136.] Wootan, Tr. II at 78-79.

[137.] Byrd-Bredbenner, Tr. I at 262; Montgomery, Tr. II at 77; Miller, Tr. II at 78.

138. Association of National Advertisers Comment at 6.

139. Berlind, Tr. I at 260; Leach, Tr. I at 161.

140. Donahue, Tr. I at 162, 194 (describing McDonald's "What I Eat and What I Do" and other balanced lifestyle ad campaigns); *See also* "McDonald's Launches New Worldwide Balanced, Active Lifestyles Public Awareness Campaign," McDonald's Press Release (March 8, 2005).

141. Kellogg Comment at 5.

142. The Public Health Advocacy Institute (PHAI) Comment at 3.

143. PBH Presentation at 4; Brugler at 223-4; PBH Press Release, "All for Good Cause: PBH Takes Home Top Health Marketing Honor" (June 20, 2005).

144. One participant had several other suggestions for in-store promotions that would encourage children to buy healthier products, such as shelf markers that flag healthy products for children, special displays of healthy products, and incentives or premiums that allow children to earn points and redeem prizes like sports equipment. Nancy Childs Comment at 1.

145. PBH Presentation at 10; Brugler, Tr. I at 225.

146. http://www.kidnetic.com.

147. Kraft, for instance, has announced that by the end of 2006, only its more nutritious "Sensible Solutions" products will appear on Kraft websites that primarily reach children ages 6 11. *See* http://www.kraft.com/newsroom/09152005.html.

148. Harris, Tr. I at 239; *see also* Society for Public Health Education Comment (community based approaches are proven effective).

149. ACFN Comment; GMA Comment at 4-5.

150. GMA Comment at 7. Examples include: Kellogg's partnership with "Girls on the Run," a 12-week after-school program for girls ages 8 to 11 years that is active in 100 cities and focuses on running games, workouts, and a 5-kilometer race (Harris, Tr. I at 220); "Triple Play," an after- school health and wellness program with the Boys and Girls Clubs of America that has been funded for five years by Kraft and Coca-Cola (Kraft Comment at 4); Kraft's "Salsa Sabor y Salud," a healthy lifestyle program for Latino families and children ages 3 to12 (Kraft Comment at 4 and GMA Survey at 14); General Mills "Champions" program, which gives grants to community-based groups to develop programs to encourage balanced diet and physical activity (GMA Survey at 14); and McDonald's "Go Active America" challenge, a 36-day program going to communities across the country to educate about nutrition and fitness, and distribute step counters along with adult "happy meals" with salad and water (Donahue, Tr. I at 161).

[151.] American Beverage Association Press Release (Aug. 6, 2005), *available at* http://www.ameribev.org/pressroom/2005_vending.asp.

[152.] *Id.*; Rodgers, Tr. I at 152.

[153.] Rodgers, Tr. I at 153.

[154.] CIFC Comment (June 7, 2005) at 12-13.

[155.] One example of a program that will monitor progress is The Kids Fitness Challenge, a pilot program in elementary, middle, and high schools, funded by corporate donors and supported by CDC and the President's Council on Fitness. The program will take a comprehensive approach to addressing childhood obesity in schools by offering fresh fruits and vegetables, healthy snacking in vending machines, and physical activity programs. The impact of the program will be monitored through children's test scores, physical fitness, attendance, and discipline. Wordin, Tr. II at 99.

[156.] *GAO Report on Commercial Activities in Schools*, GAO-04-8 10 (Aug. 2004) at 5, Table 1.

[157.] *Foods and Beverages Sold Outside of the School Meal Programs: Fact Sheet*, School Health Policies and Programs Study 2000, Centers for Disease Control and Prevention (98% of high schools, 74% of middle schools, and 43% of elementary schools have vending machines, school stores, canteens, or snack bars where students can purchase food and beverages independent of the USDA-supervised school meals programs).

[158.] "Foods Sold in Competition with USDA School Meal Programs: A Report to Congress," USDA, Food and Nutrition Service (Jan. 12, 2001) at 4, *available at* http://www.fns.usda.gov/cnd/Lunch/CompetitiveFoods/report_congress. htm. More recently, a 2004 CDC study reported "although the majority of schools offered some nutritious foods and beverages [outside of the USDA-supervised meal programs], the majority of schools also offered less nutritious choices. "Competitive Foods and Beverages Available for Purchase in Secondary Schools - - Selected Sites, United States" (2004), 54 MMWR Weekly 917 (Sept. 23, 2005) (hereinafter "Competitive Foods"). Similarly, the 2000 CDC study showed that less healthy snacks and drinks dominate the offerings. Soft drinks, high-fat salty snacks and baked goods, and candy are more widely available than healthier choices like 100% fruit juices, bottled water, milk, and low-fat snacks and baked goods. CDC 2000 Study. A more recent CSPI survey suggests offerings have not improved. The 2004 survey of 1,420 vending machines in 521 middle and high schools found that 70% of the beverage options were drinks with added sugar such as soda, juice drinks, iced tea, and sports drinks, and 80% of snack options were candy, chips, and sweet baked goods. *Dispensing Junk: How School Vending Undermines Efforts to*

Feed Children Well, Center for Science in the Public Interest (May 2004) at 4. These reports have also suggested that the prevalence of foods that are high in calories and low in nutrition contributes to children's poor eating habits and to childhood obesity. USDA/FNS 2001 Report at 4; *see also Dispensing Junk*, CSPI (May 2004).

[159.] Berlind, Tr. I at 211; Kraft Presentation at Slide 3.

[160.] Rodgers, Tr. I at 153. Some participants pointed out, and beverage companies acknowledged, that the soft drink manufacturers may lack the authority to ensure compliance with their nutritional standards by the regional bottlers that typically contract with the schools. CIFC Comment (June 7, 2005) at 9; Pepsi Presentation.

[161.] Leach, Tr. I at 218 and Pepsi Presentation.

[162.] American Beverage Association Press Release (Aug. 16, 2005), http://www. ameribev.org/pressroom/2005_vending.asp.

[163.] As one example, the American Beverage Association proposal to limit high school soft drink (including full-calorie juice drinks with less than 5% juice) sales to 50% or less of offerings may not lead to significant improvements, if any, from existing ratios. The 2004 CSPI survey suggests that, on average, levels are already below 50%. Of 1,420 vending machines in 251 schools, 39% of high school vending machines slots were for regular soft drinks and 6% for diet soft drinks, well under the 50% recommended by the ABA policy. CSPI 2004 Vending Machine Survey at 5, Table 1. Also, because the policy allows companies to wait until existing beverage contracts expire, implementation may be slow.

[164.] CIFC Comment (June 7, 2005) at 7-9.

[165.] Ross Getman Comment at 2.

[166.] CIFC Comment (June 7, 2005) at 7.

[167.] Some participants cited sports drinks as an example of a drink with high sugar content and minimal nutrition that meets nutritional standards for sale in schools under some company policies. CIFC Comment (June 7, 2005) at 9.

[168.] Some argue that older children are more vulnerable to marketing and sales in schools because they have more money and opportunity to purchase foods without their parents' knowledge or involvement. Wootan, Tr. II at 72-3. Furthermore, the USDA has determined that children in their middle and high school years have less nutritious diets. USDA found, for instance, that girls, ages 14 to 18, have especially low intakes of fruits and dairy products and more than two-thirds of them have a diet that exceeds recommended intake of total fat and saturated fat. Teenage boys are especially heavy consumers of soda, with over a third consuming more than three servings a day. USDA/FNS 2001 Report at 4.

[169.] McKinnon, Tr. I at 258.

[170.] "Competitive Foods" at 917.

[171.] *GAO Report on Commercial Activities in Schools*, GAO-04-8 10 (Aug. 2004) at 10.

[172.] Child Nutrition and WIC Reauthorization Act of 2004, Pub. L. No. 108-265, § 204, 118 Stat. 729 (2005).

[173.] *See* USDA Wellness Policy Requirements, *available at* http://www.fns. usda.gov/tn/Healthy/wellness_policyrequirements.html.

[174.] *See* IOM, Food and Nutrition Board, *Nutrition Standards for Foods in Schools*, project overview available at http://www.iom.edu/SchoolFoods2006.

[175.] Reeves, Tr. I at 173.

[176.] Dr. Dietz, of CDC, observed that there is a direct relationship between a child having a television in his room and the amount of television he watches. Dietz, Tr. I at 54.

[177.] Reeves, Tr. I at 173.

[178.] Arthur, Tr. I at 270.

[179.] *Id.*; Combating Childhood Obesity: Selling Health & Wellness to Families, Ad Council presentation, July 14, 2005, *available at* http://www.ftc.gov/bcp/ workshops/foodmarketingtokids/presentations/harthur.pdf.

[180.] Awareness of the Small Step messages increased from 79% to 86%. Arthur, Tr. I at 272.

[181.] The number of Hispanics that agreed that small changes in your eating habits and physical activities can have an impact on your weight and health increased from 56% to 63%. Arthur, Tr. at 272-273.

[182.] Id.; *see also* Combating Childhood Obesity: Selling Health & Wellness to Families, Ad Council presentation, July 14, 2005, *available at* http://www. ftc.gov/bcp/workshops/foodmarketingtokids/presentations/harthur.pdf.

[183.] The coalition is being supported by the Robert Wood Johnson Foundation and draws upon food and beverage companies such as Coca-Cola, Subway, Pepsi, and Kraft, as well as other corporate marketers, the media, non-profits organizations, and government agencies to implement a unified communications strategy. The Ad Council, *Ad Council Announces Collaboration to Combat Childhood Obesity "Coalition for Healthy Children,"* News Release, July 13, 2005.

[184.] *Id.*

[185.] Marketing agencies Strottman International and McCann Erickson also assisted the Ad Council with this research. *Id.* The messages developed for parents include, "Playing with your kids, the best exercise of all;" "Is your kid eating a home run or a strike out?" "Keep portions in check – size matters." Messages for children include, "Are you eating a home run or a strike out?" "Sitting around is for wimps;" "Being stuffed only makes sense if you're a turkey." Arthur, Tr. I at 276; *see also* Ad Council presentation, *available at* http://www.ftc.gov/bcp/workshops/foodmarketingtokids/presentations/harthur.pdf

[186.] Ad Council is partnering with Yankelovich, a marketing and consulting organization that provides marketing and consumer research, for the on-going study. Arthur, Tr. I at 274.

[187.] Daboub, Tr. I at 292; Press release announcing campaign, Nov. 19, 2003, *available at* http://www.univision.net/corp/en/pr/Washington_1 9112003-1.html.

[188.] Kotler, Tr. I 285-289; *see also* The Healthy Habits for Life Initiative at Sesame Workshop, Kotler Presentation, July 14, 2005, *available at* http://www.ftc.gov/bcp/workshops/foodmarketingtokids/presentations/jkotler.pdf.

[189.] *See* "'C' is for Citrus as Sunkist and Sesame Workshop Announce Healthy Habits for Life Partnership," Sesame Workshop Press Release, Nov. 7 (2005).

[190.] *See* http://www.adcouncil.org/campaigns/healthy_lifestyles/ for links to Sesame Workshop PSAs.

[191.] Rideout, Tr. I at 306.

[192.] Arthur, Tr. I at 270-7 1; *see also* Combating Childhood Obesity: Selling Health & Wellness to Families, Ad Council presentation, July 14, 2005, *available at* http://www.ftc.gov/bcp/workshops/foodmarketingtokids/presentations/harthur.pdf.

[193.] Nickelodeon Comment at 1 (June 8, 2005).

[194.] Smalls, Tr. I at 283; *see also* Nickelodeon Comment at 1.

[195.] Nickelodeon donated $600,000 in grants to communities in all 50 states through this initiative during 2004 and 2005 and is doubling the amount this year. *Id.*

[196.] Information about the full scope of the campaign is available on the Alliance for Healthier Generation website at www.healthiergeneration.org.

[197.] Rideout, Tr. I at 294-96.

[198.] Reeves, Tr. I at 176.

[199.] Rideout, Tr. I at 294.

[200.] *Id.*

[201.] *Id.*

[202.] *Id.*

[203] Rideout, Tr. I at 296; *see* http://www.ftc.gov/bcp/workshops/ foodmarketingtokids/ for link to video clip of commercials from Rideout presenatation.

[204] *Id.*

[205] For example, when pictures of broccoli and chocolate were offered as choices, the vast majority of kids – 78% – chose the chocolate over broccoli. However, when an image of Elmo was placed next to the picture of broccoli, many more children chose broccoli – 50% picked broccoli with Elmo as opposed to 22% without Elmo. Elmo had a similar effect on children's chocolate choices. Those choosing chocolate increased to 89% with Elmo, from 78% without Elmo. Kotler, Tr. I at 289-291; The Healthy Habits for Life Initiative at Sesame Workshop, Kotler Presentation, July 14, 2005, *available at* http://www.ftc.gov/bcp/workshops/foodmarketingtokids/presentations/jkotler.p df, at 12-17.

[206] Smalls, Tr. I at 282-83.

[207] *Id.*

[208] *See*, Melanie Warner, *Influencing Young Diets*, N.Y. Times, Dec. 16, 2005 (Business Section).

[209] Rideout, Tr. I at 307.

[210] Carmona, Tr. II at 13.

[211] Grier, Tr. I at 104.

[212] *Id.* at 105; *see also* Dietz, Tr. I at 52 and slide entitled Screen Media Exposure by Ethnicity, available at http://www.ftc.gov/bcp/workshops/ foodmarketingtokids/presentations/ wdietz.pdf.

[213] Dietz, Tr. I at 52.

[214] *Id.*

[215] *See* The California Endowment, "Food and Beverage Industry Marketing Practices Aimed at Children: Developing Strategies for Preventing Obesity and Diabetes" (Nov. 2003) (hereinafter "California Endowment Paper") at 8, available at http://www.calendow.org/reference/publications/pdf/disparities/at 13; Grier, Tr. I at 106. Dr. Grier reported that food companies also have developed customized products for ethnic minority youth. Some marketers have developed sweeter fruit-flavored beverages to appeal to the tastes of black and Hispanic children. *Id.* at 107.

[216] Grier, Tr. I at 105.

[217] Grier, Tr. I at 123.

[218] Grier, Tr. I at 104.

[219] Grier, Tr. I at 105.

[220] *See* California Endowment Paper at 14.

221. Grier, Tr. I at 105.

222. Sutherland, Tr. I at 167.

223. *Id.*

224. *Id.*

225. *Id.*

226. Sutherland, Tr. I at 168-69.

227. Powell, Tr. I at 183.

228. The increase in the households consuming Honey Nut Cheerios occurred between 2001 and 2002. General Mills Comment at 7.

229. Sutherland, Tr. I at 191.

230. *See, e.g.*, Grier, Tr. I at 103-07; Reeves, Tr. I at 179-80; Sutherland, Tr. I at 180; Carmona, Tr. II at 13.

231. *See, e.g.*, Reeves, Tr.I at 172-178.

232. Daboub, Tr. I at 311.

233. *Id.*

234. BET is the nation's leading television network providing entertainment, music, news and public affairs programming for the African-American audience. Popular shows include *College Hill, Club Comicview, Bobby Jones Gospel, Soul Food* and *106 & Park: BET's Top 10 Live*, none of which are intended for young children. Additional information regarding BET *available at* http://www.viacom.com/view_brand.jhtml?inID=7&sectionid=2.

235. Juzang, Tr. I at 302-303.

236. Grier, Tr. I at 123-124; Daboub, Tr. I at 306.

237. Grier, Tr. I at 106-107.

238. Majoras, Tr. I at 14.

239. *See* Leary, Tr. II at 22, 28.

240. CARU is financed by the children's advertising industry, while NAD/NARB, the self- regulatory body that reviews general advertising, not directed to children, derives its sole source of funding from membership fees paid to the Council of Better Business Bureaus. For a listing of CARU supporters, see http://www.caru.org/support/supporters.asp.

241. CARU Comment at 1.

242. The CARU Guides contain a wide range of principles and guidelines that restrict advertising claims for products, several of which specifically apply to food and beverage advertising. For example, the guidelines require advertisers not to mislead children about the nutritional benefits of a product, to depict appropriate amounts of a product for the situation portrayed, not to portray snacks as substitute for meals, and to show mealtime products in the context of a balanced diet.

[243.] GMA Comment, Appendix D.

[244.] *See, e.g., ABC Television Network Advertising Standards and Guidelines* (on file with the Commission) at 18 ("commercials for snack products may not recommend or suggest indiscriminate and/or immoderate use of the product"). *See also* Nickelodeon Comment at 2. In describing steps implemented to date, Nickelodeon described how it had: "(s)upplemented existing Children's Advertising Review Unit (CARU) guidelines and used our Board membership to prod for more self-assessment and further movement on the self-regulatory front. Specific Nickelodeon efforts include stipulating that ads for food should not condone excessive consumption; should illustrate portion sizes appropriate to the setting portrayed; and depict children in a manner that suggests that they are in control of their behavior."

[245.] *See* Hawkes Comment at 4. "Television advertising is covered by the ICC International Code of Advertising Practice (1997). According to the code, advertising should not be deceptive nor mislead, and should be clearly recognizable as advertising (ICC, 1997). The part of the code specific to children states that advertising should not: exploit the inexperience or credulity of children; mislead them about the nature of the product; have the effect of harming them mentally, physically or morally; nor make them feel inferior to their peers."

[246.] *See, e.g.*, Kellogg Comment at 8; Kraft Comment, at 3.

[247.] "Copy, sound and visual presentations should not mislead children about product or performance characteristics. Such characteristics may include, but are not limited to ... nutritional benefits." *See* CARU Guides at 4, reprinted in Appendix B [CARU gave the following example of an inquiry applying this guide: "*Advertising and packaging for Unilever's Popsicle JuicePops contained a statement, real fruit juice pops. CAR U determined that children might think they were 100 percent juice when they were about 30 percent and the advertiser eliminated the claim from both advertising and packaging.*" Lascoutx, Tr. II at 37-38] "Snack foods should be clearly depicted as such, and not as substitutes for meals." *See* CARU Guides at 5, reprinted in Appendix B.

[248.] "The amount of product featured should be within reasonable levels for the situation depicted." *See* CARU Guides at 5, reprinted in Appendix B [CARU gave the following example of an inquiry applying this guide: "*A commercial for Pringles showed four friends eating out of multiple six-serving containers of Pringles crisps. The advertiser agreed not to continue running the spot during children's programming.* CARU Comment at 5]; "Children should not be urged to ask parents or others to buy products." *See* CARU Guides at 5, reprinted in Appendix B.

[249.] "Program personalities, live or animated, should not be used to sell products, premiums or services in or adjacent to programs primarily directed to children in which the same personality or character appears." *See* CARU Guides at 8, reprinted in Appendix B.

[250.] CARU gave the following example of how it has applied its guide addressing the depiction of foods in advertising in a way that encourages good nutritional practices. *"An ad for an online promotion for Heinz Bagel Bites contained the line, the more you scarf, the more you can win. CARU believed this encouraged over-consumption of a snack food and the advertiser removed the line from its ads and its website."* Lascoutx, Tr. 11 at 39. ABC has a provision requiring disclosure in connection with the advertising of breakfast foods: "Each commercial for breakfast type products must include a simultaneous audio and video reference to the role of the product within the framework of a balanced diet." ABC Television Network Advertising Standards and Guidelines, at 18.

[251.] CARU Comment at 3.

[252.] *Id.*

[253.] NARC issued its report in response to a request from the Grocery Manufacturers of America to highlight for the public the actions taken by CARU against industry ads that violated the CARU Guides. National Advertising Review Council, *White Paper: Guidance for Food Advertising Self-Regulation* (2004) ("NARC White Paper"). More recently, CARU reports that, since January 2003, there have been 253 individual ads or websites that CARU recommended be modified or discontinued. CARU Comment at 3.

[254.] In 1991, CARU adopted an "Expedited Procedure" that enabled inquiries to be handled on an informal basis when advertisers established that the advertising was substantiated within ten business days of the commencement of a CARU inquiry, or made changes to the advertising within that period. Although CARU did not write formal opinions on such inquiries, it did publish short summaries. See NARC White Paper at 32-3 3. NARC abolished the informal inquiry process in 2004.

[255.] Of the 46 inquiries concerning food advertising announced on the CARU website for the period of 2000-2005, 15 concerned online privacy. Ten more concerned the promotion of sweepstakes. (Staff analysis).

[256.] Referrals to the FTC are rare. CARU notes that since 2003, there has been one referral to the Commission concerning a company that allegedly breached the CARU Guides provisions on protecting children's privacy while online. That referral lead to an FTC investigation and law enforcement action. *See United*

States v. UMG Recordings, Inc., Civ. Act, No. CV-04- 1050 JFW (Ex) (C.D. Cal. Feb. 18, 2003).

257. "The system...relies on compliance and fear of negative publicity – CARU have no sanction to fine or withdraw the advertisement, but if necessary, they can refer the case to the FTC." Hawkes Comment at 5.

258. Kraft Comment at 2.

259. Wootan, Tr. II at 50.

260. "(T)he advertising industry's thirty-year experiment with self-regulation has failed. Children see more marketing in more venues than ever before and much of this marketing is for unhealthy food ... Merely tweaking the existing system of self-regulation is not the answer." CCFC Comment at 1.

261. PHAI Comment at 2.

262. Harkin, Tr. I at 32.

263. *See, e.g.*, Attachment to PHAI Comment at 10-13. CARU disagreed, saying that it had looked at almost all of those campaigns, and found that the ads either did not violate the guides or were placed in media not directed to children. Staff conversation with Elizabeth Lascoutx, Aug. 31, 2005. Another commenter similarly suggested that certain ad campaigns violated GMA's advertising guidelines, CIFC Comment (June 7, 2005) at 2-4.

264. CCFC Comment at 6.

265. Miller, Tr. II at 73. "I think you have to expand it to more than just marketing. ... when they were talking about TV ads decreasing, if that, in fact is true, we're not talking then about marketing, and that's what I think is changing. You're talking about branded environments, you're talking about the advergames, you're talking about product placement, on and on and on and on, viral marketing as Kathy mentioned. ... it has to be expanded to include new interactive technology." *But see* Promotion Marketing Association ("PMA") Comment at 6. "We urge the agencies to reject inappropriate bans on particular advertising methods that may be unpopular with certain segments of the public interest community."

266. Molpus, Tr. II at 129. The GMA proposal is set out in Appendix C. Note that the NARC's definition of "national advertising" appears to cover advertising regardless of the medium.

267. *See supra* note 47.

268. *Id.* at 128-30.

269. For such concerns, see Harkin, Tr. I at 32. One industry member expressed a similar concern about the need for more effective enforcement. As Kellogg indicated in its comment, "to the extent that any company engages in repeat

violations involving the same principles or issues, [we] support[] referral to the FTC for additional action." Kellogg Comment at 12.

[270.] Berlind, Tr. I at 259.

[271.] CIFC Comment (Aug. 12, 2005) at 9.

[272.] *Id.*

[273.] *See* "CARU Launching Complete Review of Children's Advertising Guidelines," CARU News, Press Release (Feb. 6, 2006).

[274.] Wootan, Tr. II at 52-54.

[275.] *Id.* at 54.

[276.] *Id.* at 52-53.

[277.] "CARU was created to ensure that advertising directed to children is truthful, accurate, and appropriate for its intended audience. It was not established to be the arbiter of what products should or should not be manufactured, sold, or marketed to children, or to decide what foods are 'healthy,' or to tell parents or children what they should or shouldn't buy." CARU Comment at 4.

[278.] Wootan, Tr. II at 52.

[279.] Snyder, Tr. II at 77: "what's the consensus that these are the right nutritional standards? ... would the government set these standards? I don't think the government's going to do that. I don't think the government should do that." *See also* ADA comment at 3. "Several groups, with the best of intentions, have offered what appear on the surface to be logical, straightforward, obvious, and simple solutions to this complex problem. Yet, implementation of these solutions as policy may result in unintended consequences. Simple solutions to complex problems are generally wrong. .... Do we have evidence that restricting the advertising of certain foods really make a difference in the foods consumed at home?"

[280.] CARU Comment at 4. In fact, products that are part of Kraft's "Sensible Solutions" program are selected following a similar approach to the one set out in the CSPI Proposal. *See* Wootan, Tr. II at 90.

[281.] Wootan, Tr. II at 79: "(S)tates have regulations with nutrition standards for food sales and marketing in schools. The Federal Government has some standards around school meals .... Kraft has a model that can be looked to. PepsiCo has some nutrition standards for its marketing practice."

[282.] Montgomery, Tr. II at 77; Miller, Tr. II at 78.

[283.] One group commented that it could support the CSPI Proposal only if it were enforced by government, and then only if it applied to all food and beverage products marketed to children because even when companies pitch more healthy branded food to children they encourage them to get in the habit of making food choices based on factors that have nothing to do with nutritional qualities – and often not even on taste – but rather on packaging, premiums, contests, brand licensing and celebrity tie-ins. CCFC Comment at 2 ("any legitimate conversation about marketing ... must include the point of view that government regulation, not self regulation, is the best way to minimize the negative effect that advertising and marketing have on the health and well-being of children"); *see also* CIFC Comment (June 7, 2005) at 14 ("Given the overwhelming evidence that the food and beverage industries cannot be trusted to self-regulate, CIFC does not endorse any policy proposal that would allow them to do so. We have tried that approach and it has failed, miserably.").

[284.] Hebebrand, Tr. II at 97.

[285.] *See, e.g.,* Berlind, Tr. II at 166; Shifrin, Tr. II at 167; Molpus, Tr. II at 168.

[286.] On February 6, 2006, CARU announced that it will be convening members of the children's advertising industry to launch a complete review of the CARU Guides. According to CARU, the review project will "incorporate the work underway to examine interactive online games, paid product placement in children's television and the appropriate use of third-party licensed characters." *Supra* note 265.

In: TV, Food Marketing and Childhood Obesity   ISBN 978-1-60692-196-8
Editor: Jason Y. Cartere, pp. 95-210   © 2009 Nova Science Publishers, Inc.

Chapter 2

TV ADVERTISING IN 1977 AND 2004 INFORMATION FOR THE OBESITY DEBATE[*]

*Debra J. Holt, Debra M. Desrochers,
Pauline M. Ippolito and Christopher R. Kelley*

ABSTRACT

Obesity has become a major health concern in the U.S. and other countries as overweight and obesity rates have increased markedly since the early 1980s. The rise in children's obesity is a particular concern, because overweight children are more likely to become overweight adults, and because obese children are likely to suffer from associated medical problems earlier in life.

Food marketing is among the postulated contributors to the rise in obesity rates. Food marketing to children has come under particular scrutiny because children may be more susceptible to marketing and because early eating habits may persist. Some researchers report that children's exposure to television advertising has been increasing along with the rise in children's obesity rates.

This chapter presents a comprehensive analysis of the exposure of children, ages 2–11, to television advertising based on copyrighted Nielsen

---

[*] This is a staff report of the Bureau of Economics of the Federal Trade Commission. The views expressed in this report are those of the staff and do not necessarily represent the views of the Federal Trade Commission or any individual Commissioner.

Monitor-Plus/Nielsen Media Research audience data from the 2004 television programming season. The detailed data covers the individual advertisements shown during four weeks of national and local ad-supported programming and includes paid commercials, public service announcements, and promotions for television programming. These data are projected to annual estimates.

Thirty years ago similar assessments of children's television advertising were done for the Federal Trade Commission's 1978 Children's Advertising Rulemaking. Since these research reports were done before the rise in children's obesity, they provide a baseline to measure changes in children's exposure to television advertising.

Since the late 1970s, other marketing has likely changed and new forms of marketing have emerged, including Internet-based advertising techniques. This chapter does not cover these marketing activities, but the FTC is in the process of conducting another study to attempt to gauge the extent of all forms of marketing to children.[1]

This chapter can also be used to measure future changes in children's exposure to television advertising as industry, parents, and children react to these health concerns.

Summary of Major Findings for 2004

Children's Exposure to Television Advertising

In 2004 we estimate that children ages 211 saw about 25,600 television advertisements. In this study, advertisements include paid ads, promotions for other programming, and public service announcements. Of these 25,600 ads, approximately 18,300 were paid ads and most of the remaining 7,300 ads were promotions for other programming. The average ad seen by children was about 25 seconds long. Thus, children saw about 10,700 minutes of TV advertising in 2004. For comparison, adults saw approximately 52,500 ads and 22,300 minutes of advertising.

Our estimates differ from other published estimates of children's exposure to television advertising; one widely cited estimate, that children see around 40,000 ads per year, is more than 50 percent higher than ours. Our estimates are based on very detailed data not available to most researchers. Most published estimates are based on aggregate estimates of the amount of time children watch televi- Exposure to TV Advertising sion, combined with counts of ads aired per hour

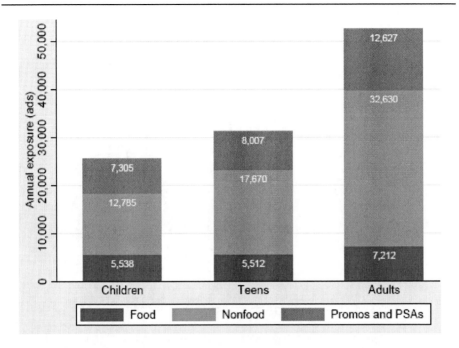

Figure ES.1. Exposure to TV Advertising.

on selected samples of TV programming. This approach can be accurate as long as the component estimates are accurate representations of children's viewing habits. But our results indicate, for instance, that ad-supported television accounts for only 70 percent of children's TV viewing in 2004, and children get much of their advertising exposure from prime time and other nonchildren's programming. These and related issues must be reflected in the component estimates for such aggregate estimates to be accurate.

Amount of Time Children Spend Viewing Ad-Supported Television

We estimate that in 2004 children 2–11 watched about two and one-quarter hours of ad-supported television per day, for a total of 16 hours per week, about 70 percent of their total television viewing time, about 23 hours per week. Teens, ages 12–17, watched about two and one-half hours of ad-supported television daily. Adults watched nearly four and one-quarter hours daily, almost twice as much as children, and this accounts for most of adults' greater ad exposure.

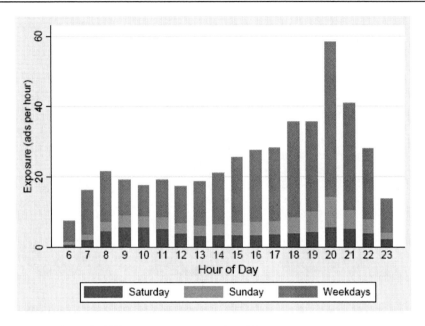

Figure ES.2. Time of Children's Exposure to Advertising.

When Children are Exposed to Ads

We find considerable dispersion in when children accumulated their ad exposure. Saturday morning between 8 am and noon was an important contributor to children's ad exposure, but was only 4.3 percent of the total. Sunday morning contributed 2.5 percent. Evenings between 8 pm and 12 am contributed nearly 29 percent of children's total ad exposure. The time between 4 pm and 8 pm contributed another 26 percent of the total. Prime-time viewing peaked around 8 pm and was the primary time when ad exposure from broadcast programming exceeded that from cable programming. These patterns of ad exposure have important implications for studies that sample children's programming in an effort to produce broad estimates of children's ad exposure, and they help to explain some of the differing results found in the research literature.

Children's Exposure to Food Advertising

Children 2–11 saw approximately 5,500 food ads in 2004, 22 percent of all ads viewed. The leading categories of food advertising seen by children include Restaurant and Fast Food (5.3 percent of total ad exposure); Cereal (3.9 percent; Highly Sugared Cereals are 85 percent of this category); Desserts and Sweets (3.5 percent); Snacks (1.9 percent); Sweetened Drinks

(1.7 percent); Dairy (1.4 percent); and Prepared Entrees (0.9 percent). All other food categories combined are 3.1 percent of ad exposure.

We also group shows according to whether the children's share of the audience is at least 20 percent (family shows) or at least 50 percent (children's shows). Food advertising is a larger share of children's advertising exposure as child share increases — from 22 percent of ad exposures on all shows to 32 percent on children's shows. The proportion of children's ad exposure is higher on children's shows for all of the food categories listed above, except for Restaurant and Fast Food ads. Children get nearly 80 percent of their Cereal ad exposure on children's shows and about one-third of their Sweetened Drink and Restaurant and Fast Food advertising there. The other food categories are between these extremes.

Sedentary Entertainment Dominates other Ads Seen by Children

Seventy-eight percent of the ads children saw in 2004 were for nonfood products. The top three nonfood product categories were Promotions for television programming (28 percent), Screen/Audio Entertainment (7.8 percent), and Games, Toys and Hobbies (7.5 percent). Together these three categories of sedentary entertainment products amounted to 43 percent of children's ad exposure, approximately double the number of food ads seen by children.

Children got approximately 85 percent of their Games, Toys and Hobbies ad exposure on children's shows, as well as 44 percent of their Screen/Audio Entertainment exposure, and 33 percent of their Promotions exposure. Together these three categories constituted 85 percent of children's nonfood ad exposure from children's shows.

Children's TV Viewing is Concentrated on Cable

Cable programming was a major source of children's television viewing and ad exposure in 2004. Sixty-one percent of children's ad exposure and 72 percent of their food ad exposure was from cable programming. For children's programming, the concentration was even higher; 96.5 percent of all children's ad exposure from children's shows and 97.6 percent of their food ad exposure from children's shows was from cable programming.

Changes in Children's Exposure to Advertising between 1977 and 2004

Children's Exposure to Paid Advertising has Fallen; Overall Ad Exposure Is up

Studies from the FTC's Children's Advertising Rulemaking indicate that children 211 saw about 19,700 paid ads and 21,900 ads overall in 1977. When compared to our estimates of 18,300 paid ads and 25,600 ads in 2004, we find that children's exposure to paid advertising fell by about 7 percent and exposure to all advertising rose by about 17 percent since 1977. This difference reflects the substantial increase in children's exposure to promotional ads for television programming over this time period. Children saw approximately 2 percent fewer minutes of advertising and 19 percent fewer minutes of paid advertising in 2004 than in 1977. These reductions reflect the combined impact of the reduced amount of time children spend watching ad-supported television in 2004 compared to 1977 and ads that are shorter on average.

Children's Exposure to Food Advertising has not Risen

The 1977 studies do not give a complete estimate of children's exposure to food ads, but using other data from the period we find that food ad exposure has not risen and is likely to have fallen modestly. In our primary scenario, we estimate that children saw 6,100 food ads in 1977. This suggests that children saw about 9 percent fewer food ads in 2004 than in 1977.

In 1977 ads for Cereals and for Desserts and Sweets dominated children's food ad exposure, with the Restaurant and Fast Food and the Sweetened Drinks categories also among the top categories. As seen above, in 2004 these categories were still among the top categories of food ads children saw, though Cereals and Desserts and Sweets no longer dominated. Restaurant and Fast Food ads had an increased presence, and were joined by Snacks, Dairy and Prepared Entrees as substantial sources of children's food ad exposure. Thus, the mix of food ads seen by children in 2004 is somewhat more evenly spread across these food categories than in 1977.

Children's Exposure to Ads for Sedentary Entertainment has Grown

The reduction in food advertisements seen by children has been more than compensated for by substantially increased Promotions for television programming and increased advertising for Screen and Audio Entertainment. These two categories are both larger than any food category in 2004 and exceed Games, Toys and Hobbies, which had been the top nonfood category in 1977.

Children's Ad Exposure is more Concentrated on Children's Cable Programming in 2004

Children get approximately half of their food advertising and about one-third of their total advertising exposure from programs in which children are at least 50 percent of the audience in 2004, compared to about one quarter in 1977. Ads for some food categories and for toys appear to be targeted to children.[2] Virtually all of this 2004 ad exposure on children's programming is from cable shows; in 1977, when cable programming was in its infancy, children's shows came from national broadcast and local sources.

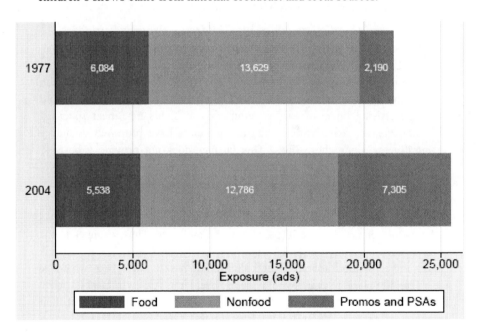

Figure ES.3. Children's Exposure: 1977 and 2004.

Discussion of Empirical Findings and Obesity

Evidence on TV Advertising's Relation to Obesity

Many commentators have suggested that marketing to children may be a significant factor in the growth of obesity in U.S. children. This hypothesis is well beyond anything we could test formally with the television advertising data analyzed here. Nonetheless, our data can shed light on aspects of this hypothesized link.

First, our data do not support the view that children are exposed to more television food advertising today. Our best estimates indicate that children's exposure to food advertising on television has fallen by about 9 percent between 1977 and 2004. Children's exposure to all paid television advertising has fallen as well.

Second, our data do not support the view that children are seeing more advertising for low nutrition foods. In both years the advertised foods are concentrated in the snacking, breakfast, and restaurant product areas. While the foods advertised on children's programming in 2004 do not constitute a balanced diet, this was the case as well in 1977, before the rise in obesity.

Evidence Related to Ad Restrictions on Children's Programming

Some have called for various restrictions on advertising to children, including a complete ban on advertising to younger children and further restrictions on the number of minutes of advertising on children's television programming. Others have called for self-regulation or legislation that would limit advertising on children's programming to foods that meet specified nutrition characteristics. Some industry members have proposed voluntary commitments along these lines. This chapter does not provide a basis to assess the likely effects of any of these approaches, or the substantial legal issues that would have to be addressed for regulation, but it does have several findings that relate to this discussion.

First, children today do get half of their food advertising from shows where children are at least 50 percent of the audience. Thus, changes to the mix of ads on children's shows could potentially have an effect on the mix and number of food advertisements that children see. This effect would be considerably larger than would have been the case in 1977, when programming was not as specialized and children did not get much of their advertising exposure from children's programs. That said, children also get half of their food advertising exposure from nonchildren's shows and food ads on those shows might increase if restrictions were placed on children's programming.

Second, our study does provide some insight on another issue that has received little attention in the public discussion: what type of advertising would likely replace the restricted food advertising, if it is replaced? The hope is that advertising for better food might increase. Beyond that, the best guidance on this question is found by looking at the other products currently advertised on children's programs, since these are the products most likely to increase their advertising if food advertising is reduced. Currently, advertisements for sedentary entertainment products outnumber food advertisements by two to one and constitute most of the other advertising on children's programming. Presumably these products would expand their advertising further, if food advertising is reduced. Whether such a shift in advertising seen by children would affect obesity in U.S. children either positively or negatively — is an open question which has received little attention.

Finally, it is worth noting that a restriction on advertising on children's programming would not fall evenly on industry participants. In 2004 broadcast networks had very few programs where children were more than 50 percent of the audience. Successful children's programming is now largely on children's cable networks. In fact, over 97 percent of food advertisements children see on children's shows are from cable programming.

Final Notes

Our study is limited to advertising on television. Television is still the medium where food advertisers spend most of their advertising dollars. In 2004 approximately 75 percent of all food advertising spending on measured media was spent on television, down from 83 percent in 1977. Many producers are exploring other advertising media and methods as television audiences become more expensive to reach. This is true for advertising to children as well. Advergaming, child-oriented producer-sponsored websites, product placements and other tieins with movies and television programming are all part of the marketing landscape, and research to quantify these efforts is only beginning.[3]

This study was conducted to provide a comprehensive assessment of the amount and type of television advertising seen by children in 2004. It has been nearly 30 years since the last evaluation of children's television ad exposure using detailed viewing data. Advertising seen by children has received considerable attention in recent years as a possible contributor to rising obesity in American children, and as a possible vehicle to help reverse that trend. Hopefully, this chapter will provide useful information to guide discussion of the issues. The chapter also provides a baseline against which to measure future changes in children's exposure to television advertising as parents, firms and children react to obesity concerns.

Table 1.1. Trends in Overweight Among Children, Adolescents, and Adults
Percent of population

Age	NHANES I 1971–1974	NHANES II 1976–1980	NHANES III 1988–1994	NHANES 1999–2000	NHANES 2001–2002	NHANES 2003–2004
2–5	5	5	7	10	11	14
6–11	4	7	11	15	16	19
12–19	6	5	11	16	17	17
20+	—	47	56	64	66	66

Source: Ogden et al. (2006) for NHANES 1999–2004; Ogden et al. (2002) for NHANES I–III for children and adolescents; and CDC (2005) for NHANES I–III for adults.

Note: Overweight defined as BMI for age at 95th percentile or higher on standard sex- and age-specific CDC growth charts for children and adolescents and BMI ≥ 25.0 for adults.

1. INTRODUCTION

Obesity has become a major health concern in the U.S. and other countries. As Table 1.1 shows, the fraction of the population that is overweight has increased markedly since the early 1980s. The rise in children's obesity is a particular concern, because overweight children are more likely to become overweight adults, and because obese children are likely to suffer from associated medical problems such as diabetes earlier in life.

Food marketing is among the postulated contributors to the rise in obesity rates. Food marketing to children has come under particular scrutiny because children may be more susceptible to marketing and because early eating habits may persist. Some researchers report that children's exposure to television advertising has been increasing along with the rise in children's obesity (e.g., IOM 2005; Hastings et al. 2003).

This chapter undertakes a comprehensive analysis of children's exposure to television advertising in 2004. We estimate that, on average, children 2–11 viewed 25,629 television ads annually. Of these 5,538 were food ads (food ads constituted 21.6 percent of all children's television ad exposure). The largest categories of food ads viewed were Restaurants and Fast Food (5.3 percent of all ads viewed), Cereal (3.9 percent), Desserts and Sweets (3.5 percent), and Snacks (1.9 percent). Children's nonfood advertising exposure was concentrated in Promotions for television programs (27.7 percent of all ads viewed), Games, Toys and Hobbies (7.5 percent), and Screen/Audio Entertainment (7.8 percent).[4]

We also examine the sources of children's advertising exposure. We find that 41.2 percent of their exposure to TV advertising comes from shows with a relatively small children's audience (fewer than one percent of the child population watching) and for which the show's audience had a small percentage of children (less than 20 percent).[5] A substantial amount of their advertising exposure, 31.3 percent, comes from shows with larger children's audiences (greater than one percent of the child population) and for which the show's audience was largely made up of children (greater than 50 percent).[6] Thus, children view 72.5 percent of their ads on two distinct types of programming — general interest or adult-oriented programming with small child audiences and programming apparently (successfully) targeted to children with a large child share and audience.

We find that 61.4 percent of children's television advertising exposure comes from cable programming. Of the cable ads children see, 35.5 percent come from general interest or adult shows with a small children's audience (less than 1 percent of the child population) while 49.0 percent come from children's programming (children are at least 50 percent of the audience) with a large child audience (greater than 1 percent of the population).

We also examine when children receive their advertising exposures. Over the average week, children are exposed to 103.5 ads during Monday through Friday prime time television viewing (8 p.m. until midnight). This results in an average of 20.7 ads per weekday viewed during prime time. In comparison, on Saturday mornings (8 a.m. until noon) children see an average of 21.1 ads.

These findings have implications for both policy and research. First, we see that changes in advertising practices on shows for which children are disproportionately represented in the audience could have a significant impact on the mix of ads that children see. Overall, 46.9 percent of children's TV ad exposure comes from shows in which at least 20 percent of the audience is children; 33.8 percent comes from shows in which at least 50 percent of the audience is children.[7]

Second, content analysis that focuses on children's programming, defined by the time of day and day of the week, is missing a significant portion of children's advertising exposure. Over an entire week children receive 28.7 percent of their exposures during prime time and only 6.8 percent on weekend mornings.

We also review and summarize reports submitted by John Abel and J. Howard Beales to the Federal Trade Commission's 1978 Children's Advertising Rulemaking (Abel 1978; Beales 1978). Since these research reports were done in

1978, before children's obesity became a serious health problem, they provide a baseline to measure changes in children's advertising exposure on TV.

We find that children's exposure to television advertising has increased somewhat (21,904 in 1977 to 25,629 in 2004) while exposure to TV food ads has not increased and has likely decreased some since 1977. Not all food categories saw a decrease in children's viewing; we find that children's exposure to ads for Restaurants, Fast Food and Snacks has increased. On the other hand, their exposure to ads for Cereal, Desserts and Sweets has declined. Exposure to ads for Games, Toys and Hobbies also fell. The categories for which exposure has increased the most are Screen/Audio Entertainment and Promotions. Children saw very few ads encouraging active pursuits, such as ads for bicycles or other sporting goods, in either period.

2. TELEVISION LANDSCAPE IN 1977 AND 2004

Before proceeding with our analysis of advertising data, we briefly describe some of the major changes in television viewing options between 1977 and 2004. These changes shape advertising viewing patterns in our data.

2.1. Broadcast Networks Dominated in 1977

In 1977, three national broadcast networks – ABC, CBS, and NBC – and their affiliated stations dominated television advertising. According to the *Economist* (1981), network affiliates accounted for 93 percent of all TV viewing in 1975. A. C. Nielsen Co. (1977, p. 12) reported that 728 commercial stations and 256 public stations were in operation at the beginning of 1977. Of the commercial stations, 83 percent were affiliated with ABC (195), CBS (198), or NBC (209). The remaining commercial stations were independent or had some affiliation with more than one network (Abel 1978, p. 1–2). According to A. C. Nielsen Co. (1977), 96 percent of households could receive four or more stations and 66 percent of households could receive seven or more stations. Only 14 percent of households were wired for cable (A. C. Nielsen Co. 1977, p. 6).

2.2. Cable and Broadcast Networks Share the 2004 Market

These three national broadcast networks remain significant players in 2004, but they compete with an increasing number of other television programming providers. ABC, CBS, and NBC affiliates captured just 28.1 percent of prime time viewing and 28.4 percent of total day viewing in 2004, down from 93 percent in 1977. Seven other national broadcast networks were monitored by Nielsen in 2004 FOX, PAX, United Paramount Network (UPN), Warner Brothers (WB), Telemundo (TEL), TeleFutura (TF), and Univision (UNI). In addition, Nielsen monitors 10 independent broadcast TV stations in the top 75 local markets.

Cable television has grown significantly in the intervening years. The Cabletelevision Advertising Bureau (CAB) reports 65 national cable networks. Cable reaches approximately 85 percent of households in the U.S. Of the 65 national cable networks in operation during 2004, 36 reached at least 70 percent of the national market (Cabletelevision Advertising Bureau 2006b,a,d). Cable attracted about one-third of all television advertising dollars.[8] Cable captured 43.9 percent of prime time and 46.5 percent of total daily viewing during the 2003–2004 programming season (Cabletelevision Advertising Bureau 2006c). While cable's overall share continues to increase, no single cable network is viewed by more than 40 percent of the population in an average week. In contrast, ABC, CBS, FOX, and NBC are all viewed by at least 70 percent of the population in an average week.[9]

2.3. Increasing Specialization and Segmentation

The growth in television providers has coincided with increasing specialization and market segmentation. More networks produce and distribute television programming; however, people are not watching more television. Adults spent about the same amount of time watching TV in 2004 as in 1977, about four hours per day, while children reduced their TV watching, from about four hours per day to about three and a quarter hours per day (of which two and a quarter hours was ad-supported TV).[10] Thus, networks face increased competition for viewers. Some networks have responded by offering programming content narrowly targeted to certain populations "Animal Planet" and "Cartoon Network," for example.

Part of the specialization in children's programming may be related to the fact that children had a greater opportunity to watch TV independently from their parents in 2004 than in 1977. The Kaiser Family Foundation found that 73 percent of 8 18 year olds and 67 percent of 8–10 year olds live in households with three or more TVs. Also, 84 percent of children 6 months to 6 years old live in households with two or more television sets (Roberts et al. 2005). Approximately 33 percent of children 6 months to 6 years old have a television in their bedroom, and for 33 percent of these, at least half of total television viewing occurs in their bedroom (Rideout and Hamel 2006). In comparison, only 45 percent of households owned more than one TV in 1977 (A. C. Nielsen Co. 1977).

With the three major networks dominating the television landscape in 1977, less specialization or market segmentation was possible. These changes as they relate to children's viewing can be seen from the relative numbers of children watching specific programs in the two periods. In 1977 more than 24 percent of all children watched the top nine network programs; more than 10 percent of all children watched the top 60 network programs (Abel 1978, Appendix C). In contrast, in 2004 no program had 10 percent of children watching. The top ranked show by child audience size in our 2004 data drew approximately 8 percent of all children ("American Idol"). Only 11 shows in our data were watched by more than 5 percent of the 2 11 population. Few shows 7 percent were watched by more than one percent of the 2–11 population.

While relatively few shows had large child audiences in 2004, many shows successfully specialized in entertaining children. We will explore these issues in detail later, but a few points are appropriate here. Many shows in 2004 had audiences where children constituted a high share of the audience. Moreover, those 2004 shows with a predominantly child audience often also had a high (for 2004) child audience size. For example, about half of the top fifty shows each month ranked by size of the child audience also had a child share greater than 50 percent. Finally, this overlap occurred primarily on cable; children constituted a large share of the audience for few broadcast programs.

So overall, the TV world of 1977, with fewer programs aimed at broad audiences, has shifted to a world with many more program choices, smaller audiences for those programs, and more specialized programming appealing to narrower segments of the audience, including the children of interest in this study.

3. TELEVISION ADVERTISING IN 2004

Children are exposed to advertisements as they watch television. The question of how many advertisements children see, and whether that number has increased substantially over time, has been a topic of considerable interest as investigators attempt to identify the major factors potentially contributing to the rise in childhood obesity in America. Thus, one of the first issues we examine for 2004 is the total number of advertisements that children see. In subsequent sections we examine when and where children get their advertising exposure in 2004, what products are featured in that advertising, and how much of that advertising comes from "children's programming." We also present some information on advertising to young children.

We investigate exposure to television advertising using a comprehensive database of advertising aired during four weeks in the 2003–2004 programming season.[11] We use copyrighted Nielsen Monitor-Plus/Nielsen Media Research data linking Nielsen audience estimates to the television advertising aired on ad-supported television during the 20032004 programming season. The data covers advertising aired during the four weeks beginning November 2, 2003, February 8, 2004, May 2, 2004, and July 4, 2004.[12] We chose these weeks in order to match the Abel and Beales 1978 studies of children's exposure to television advertising and because they occur during sweeps periods, the only times detailed local data is available. We do not know how viewing and advertising patterns in these weeks may differ from the rest of the year. However, sweeps periods are used to determine pricing for local spot ads and thus should only affect network affiliate programming, advertising, and promotions; as we will see later in this section, less than 40 percent of children's advertising exposure is from network affiliates.

The data includes all television advertisements aired during the monitored ad-supported programs. These include paid commercial advertisements, public service announcements (PSAs), and Promotions for a network's own or affiliated programming. Networks that are not ad-supported are not included in our data. Therefore we have no information on Promotions on pay cable networks or sponsorship messages such as those aired on Disney and PBS.[13] The data covers both national advertising and local spot advertising and includes nearly one million national ads and nearly five million local spot ads.[14] In addition to audience estimates for children, younger children, teens, and adults, the data includes, for each ad, information on the advertiser, the brand, the television network, the program, the time the ad aired, the ad's length, and a product code.

We use Gross Rating Points (GRPs), which represent the percentage of a given population that is estimated to be in the audience of a program or commercial, to estimate children's average exposure to advertising.[15] Multiplying the child GRP for an ad by the 2–11 population yields an estimate of the number of children who viewed that ad.

To illustrate the process of estimating annual ad exposure, consider calculating the "average" child's exposure for one day in our data. First, calculate the estimated number of children who saw each ad, as described above. Then sum over all the ads aired on all television programming over that day. The resulting figure is the total number of ads seen by all children in the U.S. that day. Finally, dividing by the 2–11 population gives the estimated number of ads the average child saw that day.[16]

To estimate the average annual exposure to television advertising, we follow the above procedure using all four weeks of our data and multiply the result by 365/28.

3.1. Children's Exposure to Advertising

Table 3.1 presents our estimates of children's exposure to TV advertising. We estimate that children ages 211 saw, on average, 25,629 television ads per year in 2004. This figure includes paid ads as well as Promos (promotions for other television programming) and PSAs (public service announcements). Young children 2–5 saw 24,939 ads per year, while older children in the group ages 6–11 saw 26,079 ads per year.[17] Average exposure to TV ads in 2004 continues to rise with age those 12–17 saw 31,188 ads per year, while those 18 years of age and over saw 52,469 ads per year. Thus adults saw more than twice as many ads as children. We will see later in this section that much of the exposure differences between age groups can be traced to differences in time spent watching television.

Table 3.1 also provides data on exposure to minutes of television advertising, in addition to numbers of ads. The two together imply that the average television ad viewed is around 25 seconds long, for all age groups.[18] We find considerable variation in ad length in 2004. Many ads are 15 second (and shorter) in length, but a considerable number of ads are longer than 30 seconds particularly one minute ads.[19]

How much Ad-supported TV do People Watch?

Our data allows us to estimate the hours per day that children, and other age groups, watch Nielsen-monitored, ad-supported television.[20] For each half-hour block of time, we calculate the average number of children watching all programming (using the GRPs for each ad in that time block). Then we can calculate the number of children-hours of TV watching over a 24-hour period by summing the number of children watching in each time block over the day. Then we divide by the population of children 2–11 to obtain the number of hours the average child watched television in that 24-hour period. This method is extended to all 4 weeks of data and averaged.

Table 3.1. Annual Exposure to TV Advertising by Children, Teens, and Adults

	All advertising		Paid advertising		Food advertising	
	Ads	Minutes	Ads	Minutes	Ads	Minutes
Children (ages 2-11)	25,629	10,717	18,324	7, 987	5,538	2,202
Younger children (ages 2 – 5)	24, 939	10,425	17,669	7,678	5, 390	2,140
Older children (ages 6 – 11)	26,079	10,908	18,750	8,189	5,635	2,242
Teens (ages 1217)	31,188	13,127	23,181	10,306	5,512	2,193
Adults (ages 18 and over)	52,469	22,271	39,842	18, 043	7,212	2,834

Source: Staff analysis of copyrighted Nielsen Media Research/Nielsen Monitor–Plus data; four weeks projected annually.

Note: Paid advertising excludes promotional advertising for a network's own or affliated shows and public service announcements.

Compare this to the more common method of estimating the average amount of children's daily television viewing. Typically a sample of children (or their parents) are each asked about the number of hours per day that they watch television. Those numbers are summed and then divided by the number of children in the sample. We instead "sample" hours and check for the number of children watching in those time blocks. Note that before the final step dividing by the number of children both methods obtain comparable figures: thetotal number of hours that all the children watched television.[21]

Table 3.2. Daily Ad-Supported TV Viewing

	Overall	Cable		Broadcast	
	Hours	Hours	%	Hours	%
Children (ages 2–11)	2:17	1:31	66.5	0:46	33.5
Younger children (ages 2–5)	2:19	1:35	68.5	0:44	31.5
Older children (ages 6–11)	2:16	1:29	65.1	0:47	34.9
Teens (ages 1217)	2:31	1:27	57.3	1:04	42.7
Adults (ages 18 and over)	4:10	1:49	43.6	2:21	56.4

Source: Staff analysis of copyrighted Nielsen Media Research/Nielsen Monitor–Plus data; four weeks projected annually.

As shown in Table 3.2 we find that, on average, children 211 watch just over two and one-quarter hours (2:17) of ad-supported TV per day. Teenagers (ages 12–17) watch just over two and one-half hours (2:31) per day, and adults watch nearly four and one-quarter hours (4:10) of ad-supported television per day. Our estimates for children's viewing time are roughly consistent with other estimates of children's viewing, given that some TV time is spent watching shows without ads, such as on public television stations or premium cable channels.[22] We find that adults watch nearly twice as much ad-supported television as children; this accounts for most of their greater exposure to television ads with the remainder due to their seeing four more ads each hour than children.[23]

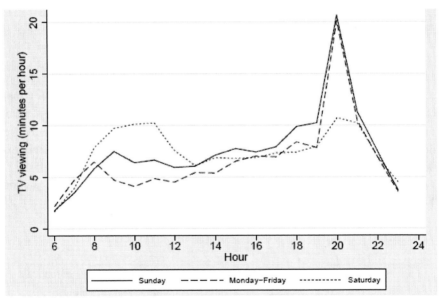

Source: Staff analysis of copyrighted Nielsen Media Research/Nielsen Monitor–Plus data; four weeks projected annually. Note: Ad-supported TV viewing averaged across weekdays.

Figure 3.1. TV Viewing Over the Day Children ages 2–11.

Children ages 2–11

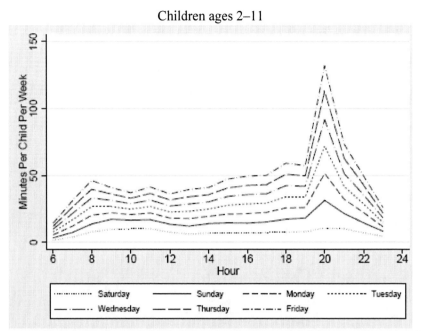

Source: Staff analysis of copyrighted Nielsen Media Research/Nielsen Monitor–Plus data;
    four weeks projected annually.
Note: Ad-supported TV viewing.

Figure 3.2. Cumulative TV Viewing Per Hour over the Week.

3.2. Time of Children's Viewing

As discussed in the previous section, children watch 2 hours and 17 minutes of ad-supported television each day on average, or about 16 hours each week (15:59). But children's viewing time, or minutes viewed per hour, varies considerably by the time of day and day of the week.

Figure 3.1 shows that for Sunday and the average weekday, there is a large spike in viewing between around 7 p.m. and 9 p.m. that peaks around 8 p.m. There is also a noticeable increase in viewing on Saturday mornings; however, minutes viewed per hour at around 8 p.m. on weeknights and Sunday is approximately twice the viewing per hour on Saturday mornings. Saturday evening viewing is comparable to Saturday morning viewing.

Figure 3.2 gives comparable information but breaks out the contribution of each weekday and stacks the time of day viewing pattern, thus showing the contribution of each hour of each day to the total week's viewing time. Over the week as a whole, children view nearly three times as much TV in the peak evening hours as in the mornings.

Children ages 2–11, cable (a) and broadcast

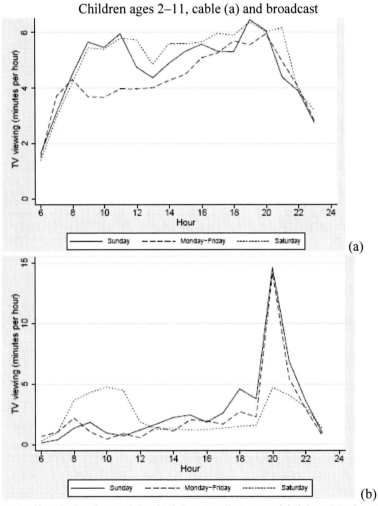

(a)

(b)

Source: Staff analysis of copyrighted Nielsen Media Research/Nielsen Monitor–Plus data; four weeks projected annually.
Note: Ad-supported TV viewing averaged across weekdays.

Figure 3.3. TV Viewing Over the Day.

Table 3.3. Percent of Advertising Exposure by Time of Day

Children ages 2–11

Time period	Sunday	Overall Weekdays	Saturday	Total
12 am – 4 am	1.0	4.5	1.1	6.5
4 am – 8 am	0.7	4.8	0.8	6.4
8 am – 12 pm	2.5	8.9	4.3	15.7
12 pm – 4 pm	2.6	11.4	2.9	16.8
4 pm – 8 pm	3.7	19.0	3.1	25.8
8 pm – 12 am	4.1	21.1	3.5	28.7
Daily total	14.5	69.7	15.8	100.0
Weekly exposure (ads per child)				491

Source: Staff analysis of copyrighted Nielsen Media Research/Nielsen Monitor–Plus data; four weeks projected annually.

As Table 3.2 indicates, 66.5 percent of children's television viewing is of cable programming. Figure 3.3 indicates that the time of viewing analysis is markedly different for cable and broadcast networks. (Note vertical scales are different.) Broadcast network viewing is responsible for virtually all the prime time peak and contributes about half of the Saturday morning peak. Except for these times, broadcast viewing is lower than cable viewing. Chil dren's viewing of cable programming is much more stable across hours of the day and days of the week. Throughout the week, except for very early morning and very late evening hours, children view cable programming approximately as much as they view broadcast networks on Saturday mornings.

Time of Advertising Exposure

We also look at children's exposure to advertising over the day and by days of the week.[24] Table 3.3 gives exposure to advertising over four-hour blocks of the day for weekdays, Saturday, and Sunday. We see that the largest share of children's daily exposure, 21.1 ads per week or 4.3 percent of weekly exposure, comes from viewing between 8 a.m. and noon on Saturdays. However, they get approximately the same share of their advertising exposure, 20.7 ads per week or 4.2 percent of weekly exposure, on the average weekday night between 8 p.m. and midnight. The same time slot on Sunday nights is also a prominent contributor – children on average see 19.9 ads per week or 4.1 percent of weekly advertising exposure. Figure 3.4 graphically presents the information in Table 3.3. It is evident that overall, weekday programming dominates children's total exposure to television advertising. Children get 21.1 percent of their ad exposure Monday through Friday between 8 p.m. and midnight; 19.0 percent of their exposure on weekdays between 4 p.m. and 8 p.m.; 11.4 percent of their exposure on weekdays between noon and 4 p.m.; and 8.9 percent of their exposure between on weekdays between 8 a.m. and noon. In total, children get 69.7 percent of their ad exposure on Monday through Friday programming.

Figure 3.4 indicates that Sunday is also a big day for ad exposure. Other than the Saturday morning 8 a.m. to noon block of time, Sunday, Saturday, and the average week day make comparable contributions to children's ad exposure. Sunday dominates Saturday in ad exposure from 4 p.m. until midnight and is close to Saturday's exposure for the noon to 4 p.m. period. Children also see more ads per time block on Sunday than the average weekday from 8 a.m. to 4 p.m. and close to the same ad exposure from 4 p.m. to midnight. Table 3.3 and Figure 3.4 illustrate that evening programming is an important contributor to children's advertising exposure throughout the week. Children get 28.7 percent of their weekly ad exposure between 8 p.m. and midnight; they get another 25.8 percent of their exposure between 4 p.m. and 8 p.m. Despite the high level of exposure to advertising on Saturday mornings, over the entire week the 8 a.m. to noon time period contributes only 15.7 percent of children's weekly advertising exposure. The afternoon time period contributes a similar amount, 16.8 percent of weekly ad exposure.

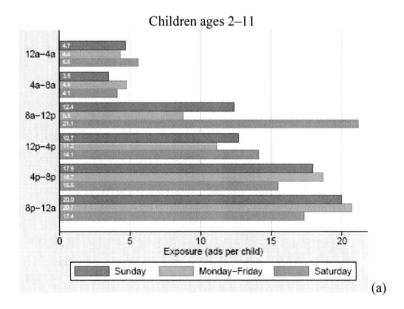

Children ages 2–11

(a)

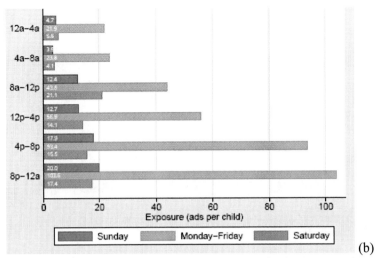

(b)

Source: Staff analysis of copyrighted Nielsen Media Research/Nielsen Monitor–Plus data; four weeks projected annually.

Note: Average exposure represents exposure on the average weekday; total exposure represents total exposure across all weekdays. Figures on different scales.

Figure 3.4. Average (a) and Total (b) Exposure to TV Advertising Over the Day.

Children ages 2–11

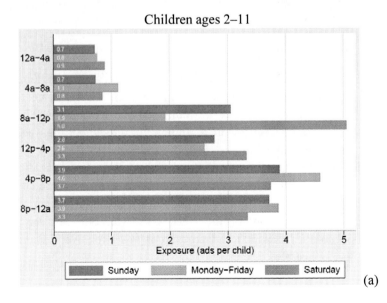

(a)

Figure 3.5. (Continued)

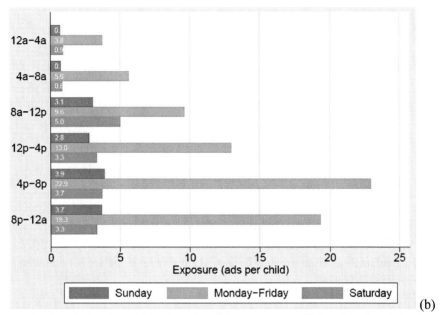

(b)

Source: Staff analysis of copyrighted Nielsen Media Research/Nielsen Monitor–Plus data; four weeks projected annually.

Note: Average exposure represents exposure on the average weekday; total exposure represents total exposure across all weekdays. Figures on different scales.

Figure 3.5. Average (a) and Total (b) Exposure to Food Advertising over the Day.

Figure 3.5 shows that food advertising follows a similar pattern, though with some move away from evening programming. Children see 4.8 percent of their food ads on Saturday mornings between 8 a.m. and noon. They get 18.2 percent of their food ad exposure between 8 p.m. and midnight throughout the week, or 3.6 percent on an average week night.

Figure 3.6 gives children's overall (food and nonfood) average ad exposure by hour for each day of the week, with the days stacked to show the cumulative contribution to overall ad exposure. The pattern is similar to that for television viewing by hour and by day of the week; however, one can see that the contribution of morning viewing to ad exposure is lower relative to that of prime time viewing; this illustrates that advertising exposure is relatively higher in prime time viewing.

Children ages 2–11

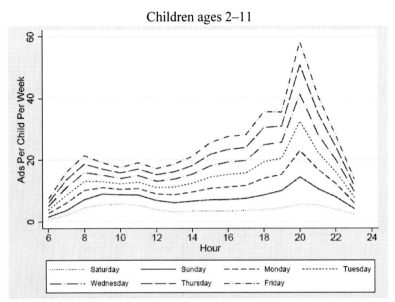

Source: Staff analysis of copyrighted Nielsen Media Research/Nielsen Monitor–Plus data; four weeks projected annually.

Figure 3.6. Cumulative Exposure to TV Advertising Per Hour over the Week.

As with children's television viewing over the day and the days of the week, their exposure to television advertising follows different patterns on cable and broadcast networks. Figure 3.7 illustrates how each hour of each day contributes to the average child's total exposure to advertising on cable and broadcast programming. It is only during the evening hours of peak viewing that weekly exposure from broadcast programming surpasses exposure from cable programming.

We see that conclusions about the nature of children's exposure to television advertising based on analyses of Saturday morning programming may be misleading, as they get only 4.3 percent of their weekly ad exposure from that time/day slot. Adding weekday after-school programming to the analysis gives a broader picture of children's exposure — together, weekdays between 4 p.m. and 6 p.m. contribute 8.4 percent of children's ad exposure. However, nearly 30 percent of children's exposure to television advertising comes on programming aired between 8 p.m. and midnight, nearly double the exposure from programming in time periods often treated as representative of children's viewing. Further, we see that patterns of viewing and ad exposure on cable networks, where 66.5 percent of their viewing takes place, are considerably different than on broadcast networks.

Children ages 2–11, cable (a) and broadcast (b)

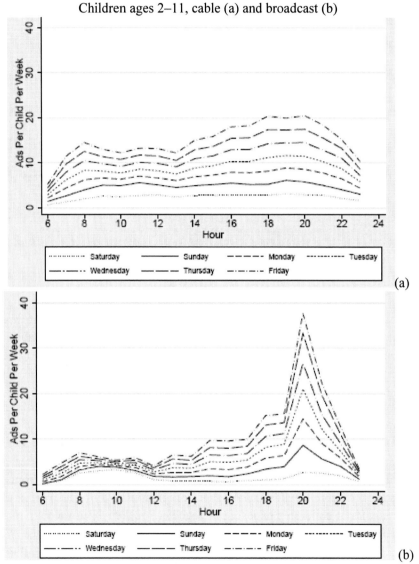

(a)

(b)

Source: Staff analysis of copyrighted Nielsen Media Research/Nielsen Monitor–Plus data; four weeks projected annually.

Figure 3.7. Cumulative Exposure to TV Advertising Per Hour Over the Week.

3.3. Product Advertising Seen by Children

The types of products advertised to children are not randomly chosen. From an economic point of view, we would expect producers to advertise products on children's programs that they believe children will either buy themselves or will have a role in choosing in the family. Moreover, children do not watch only children's programs. So their exposure to product advertising is also shaped by the mix of other programming they view.

A number of studies from the past have found that the foods advertised on children's programs have been heavily concentrated in the sweetened cereal, candy, snacks, and beverage categories (Kunkel and Gantz 1992; Kotz and Story 1994; Byrd-Bredbenner 2002). Toys have also been consistently found to be heavily advertised to children.

In this section, we provide a detailed examination of the types of product ads seen by children in 2004. We also examine how much of the advertising in various categories comes from children's programming as opposed to other types of programming.

We specifically examined 41 product categories — 28 food categories and 13 nonfood categories.[25] In order to simplify our analysis, we aggregate some of these detailed categories into fewer, and broader, product categories. After the initial presentation of the results we will use these broader product categories.

We estimate that in 2004 children ages 2–11 saw 5,538 food ads per year and 20,091 ads for other products. Table 3.4 shows, in the three left-most columns, children's average annual ad exposure in each category along with the percentage of total ad exposure that category contributes. We also show, in the three right columns, children's average annual ad exposure in each of the detailed categories.[26] This illustrates the relative contribution of each of the detailed categories. For example, Highly Sugared Cereal accounts for 84 percent of children's exposure to ads for Cereal (3.3 of the 3.9 percent total) and Candy accounts for 52 percent of children's exposure to ads for Desserts and Sweets (1.8 of the 3.5 total for the category).

The largest categories of food ads viewed by children are: Restaurants and Fast Food (5.3 percent of all ad exposure); Cereal (3.9 percent); Desserts and Sweets (3.5 percent); Snacks (1.9 percent); Sweetened Drinks (1.7 percent); and Dairy Products (1.4 percent). All other itemized (detailed) food categories contribute less than one percent of ad exposure each.

Table 3.4. Annual Exposure to TV Advertising By Product Categories

			Children 2–11		
Category	Ads	%	Detailed category	Ads	%
Cereal	993	3.9	Regular Cereal	157	0.6
			Highly Sugared Cereal	836	3.3
Desserts and Sweets	898	3.5	Candy	468	1.8
			Desserts and Dessert Ingredients	52	0.2
			Cakes, Pies and Pastries	94	0.4
			Regular Gum	104	0.4
			Cookies	166	0.6
			Ice Cream	15	0.1
Restaurants and Fast Food	1,367	5.3	Restaurants and Fast Food	1,367	5.3
Snacks	490	1.9	Appetizers, Snacks and Nuts	343	1.3
			Crackers	99	0.4
			Snack, Granola and Cereal Bars	48	0.2
Dairy Products	353	1.4	Dairy Products and Substitutes	353	1.4
Sweetened Drinks	430	1.7	Regular Carbonated Beverages	147	0.6
			Regular Non-carbonated Beverages	283	1.1
Prepared Entrees	222	0.9	Prepared Entrees	205	0.8
			Frozen Pizza	17	0.1
Other Food	786	3.1	Beer, Wine and Mixers	132	0.5
			Diet Carbonated Beverages	20	0.1
			Diet Non-carbonated Beverages	17	0.1
			Fruit Juices	51	0.2
			Sugarless Gum	25	0.1
			Canned Fruit	0	0.0
			Raisins and Other Dried Fruit	0	0.0
			Fresh Fruit	0	0.0
			Vegetables and Legumes	16	0.1
			Meat, Poultry and Fish	48	0.2
			Bread, Rolls, Waffles and Pancakes	155	0.6
			Other Food and Beverage	322	1.3
All Food Products	**5,538**	**21.6**	**All Food Products**	**5,538**	**21.6**
Games, Toys and Hobbies	1,909	7.5	Games, Toys and Hobbies	1,909	7.5
Screen / Audio	2,010	7.8	Screen / Audio Entertainment	2,010	7.8

Entertainment					
Sports and Exercise	24	0.1	Sporting Goods	23	0.1
			Exercise Equipment	1	0.0
Promos and PSAs	7,305	28.5	Promos	7,097	27.7
			PSAs	208	0.8
Other Nonfood	8,842	34.5	Dental Supplies	220	0.9
			Diets and Diet Aids	64	0.2
			Footwear	111	0.4
			Computer Hardware and Internet Services	230	0.9
			Computer Software (Non-game)	13	0.0
			Over-the-counter Medication	648	2.5
			Prescription Medication	312	1.2
			Other Nonfood Advertising	7,244	28.3
All Nonfood Products	**20,091**	**78.4**	**All Nonfood Products**		**20,091 78.4**
Total	25,629		Total		25,629

Source: Staff analysis of copyrighted Nielsen Media Research/Nielsen Monitor–Plus data; four weeks projected annually.

The largest nonfood categories we examined are: Promos and PSAs (28.5 percent of all ad exposure; of this Promos contribute 27.7 percentage points, or 97 percent of the category); Games, Toys and Hobbies (7.5 percent); and, Screen/Audio Entertainment (7.8 percent). Over-the-Counter Medications (2.5 percent) and Prescription Medications (1.2 percent) are the only other categories that contribute more than one percent of children's total advertising exposure.[27]

The Sports and Exercise category makes up only 0.1 percent of all ad exposures. In contrast, the largely sedentary product categories — Games, Toys and Hobbies, Screen/Audio entertainment, and Promos make up 43.0 percent of all children's advertising exposure.[28] Note that this is approximately double the number of food ads seen by children; food ads constitute 21.6 percent of ad exposure.

3.4. Product Ads Viewed Vary by Type of Show

We also look at how children's exposure to product ads varies over different types of shows, where shows are grouped by the proportion of children in the shows' audience.[29] This is of interest for several reasons. First, we can determine whether the product mix of ads changes as the proportion of children in the audience increases. Second, we can provide information on the potential impact of any proposed advertising restrictions that are based on the proportion of children in the audience. For example, restricted advertising on children's shows would have little impact if the children are watching general interest or adult-oriented programming in larger numbers. In the next section we examine the relationship between shows' child audience size and the proportion, or share, of children in the shows' audience.[30]

We refer to the proportion of a show's audience that is children as the child audience share. For example, a child audience share of 20 percent indicates that at least 20 percent of that show's total audience is made up of children ages 2–11.[31] We group shows according to whether the children's share of the audience is at least 20 percent (referred to as family shows) or at least 50 percent (referred to as children's shows).[32] We find that 87.7 percent of all shows have a children's audience share of less than 20 percent. Nevertheless, 47.0 percent of children's advertising exposure comes from the 12.3 percent of shows that have a children's audience share of 20 percent or more.

Table 3.5. Annual Exposure to TV Advertising by Child Share of Audience

	Children ages 2–11					
Category	All ads		Share ≥ 20%		Share ≥ 50%	
	Ads	%	Ads	%	Ads	%
Cereal	993	3.9	888	7.4	782	9.0
Desserts and Sweets	898	3.5	655	5.4	520	6.0
Restaurants and Fast Food	1, 367	5.3	656	5.5	436	5.0
Snacks	490	1.9	389	3.2	341	3.9
Dairy Products	353	1.4	271	2.3	239	2.8
Sweetened Drinks	430	1.7	234	1.9	162	1.9
Prepared Entrees	222	0.9	141	1.2	113	1.3
Other Food	786	3.1	280	2.3	198	2.3
All Food Products	5, 538	21.6	3,515	29.2	2, 792	32.2
Games, Toys and Hobbies	1, 909	7.5	1, 827	15.2	1, 629	18.8
Screen / Audio Entertainment	2, 010	7.8	1, 205	10.0	888	10.2
Sports and Exercise	24	0.1	16	0.1	12	0.1
Promos and PSAs	7, 305	28.5	3, 552	29.5	2, 474	28.5
Other Nonfood	8, 842	34.5	1, 923	16.0	877	10.1
All Nonfood Products	20, 091	78.4	8, 523	70.8	5, 881	67.8
Total	25,629		12,038		8,673	

Source: Staff analysis of copyrighted Nielsen Media Research/Nielsen Monitor–Plus data; four weeks projected annually.

Children ages 2–11

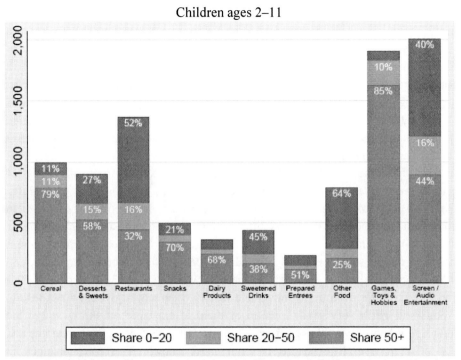

Source: Staff analysis of copyrighted Nielsen Media Research/Nielsen Monitor–Plus data;
   four weeks projected annually.
Note: Promos and PSAs and Other Nonfood Advertising omitted because they obscure
   differences of interest.

Figure 3.8. Annual Exposure to TV Advertising, Selected Categories.

As shown in Table 3.5, as the share of children in the audience increases, food advertising exposure increases from 21.6 percent on all shows, to 32.2 percent on children's shows. The proportion of ad exposure from Cereal; Desserts and Sweets; Snacks; Dairy Products; Prepared Entrees; Games, Toys and Hobbies; and Screen/Audio Entertainment all increase as the share of children in the audience increases. The contribution of Restaurants and Fast Food to ad exposure rises and then falls slightly as children's audience share increases.

Figure 3.8 further illustrates these findings.[33] It shows the estimated exposures in each depicted category along with the fraction that comes from programs with different shares of children in the audience. For instance, of the estimated 1,909 ads that children saw for Games, Toys and Hobbies, 85 percent were seen on programs where children are more than 50 percent of the audience, and only four percent are from shows where children are less than 20 percent of the audience. This data suggests that toy ads are highly targeted to children. Similar patterns are seen for Cereal and Snacks, also suggesting that ads in these categories are targeted to children. In contrast, of the 1,367 ads children saw for Restaurants and Fast Food, 32 percent are seen on children's shows while 52 percent are seen on shows where children are less than 20 percent of the audience, suggesting that children are less targeted for these products. The Sweetened Drinks category has a similar ad distribution, suggesting that children are not the primary targets for this advertising. Overall, 50 percent of children's exposure to food advertising comes from children's shows.

We have seen that children's ad exposure comes from all types of programming; Table 3.6 shows that the same is not true for teens and adults. Children get 50.4 percent of their food ad exposure from children's shows. In contrast, teens and adults get very little of their food ad exposure from children's shows — 15.4 and 3.1 percent. While not quite as pronounced, a similar pattern holds on family shows. Children get 63.5 percent of their food ad exposure, and 47.0 percent of all ad exposure, from these shows. Teens get 26.7 percent of their food ad exposure from these shows and just 17.6 percent of overall ad exposure. Adults still get a very small fraction of their ad exposure on shows where the audience is more than 20 percent children; only 6.1 percent of their food ads and 3.4 of their overall exposure is from these shows. Therefore, changes in advertising on children's shows, or even family shows, would have little effect on the advertising adults see and a moderate impact on teens' advertising exposure.

Table 3.6. Percent of Ad Viewing from Children's and Family Shows

	Children			Teens	Adults
	2–11	2–5	6–11	12–17	18 and over
Child 2–11 audience share ≥ 50%					
Food	50.4	55.1	47.5	15.4	3.1
Promos and PSAs	33.9	36.8	32.0	9.6	1.6
Other Nonfood	26.6	31.0	24.0	5.8	0.8
Total	33.8	37.9	31.3	8.5	1.3
Child 2–11 audience share ≥ 20%					
Food	63.5	66.1	61.8	26.7	6.1
Promos and PSAs	48.6	49.9	47.8	20.2	4.2
Other Nonfood	38.9	41.2	37.5	13.5	2.5
Total	47.0	49.1	45.6	17.6	3.4

Source: Staff analysis of copyrighted Nielsen Media Research/Nielsen Monitor–Plus data; four weeks projected annually.

3.5. How are Children's Audience Size and Share Related?

Examining ad exposure based on the children's audience share of programming suggests that children are being targeted with advertising for specific categories of products. This is not surprising given the number of television channels with specialized programming content that is intended to appeal to children and the types of products children are likely to purchase or influence. But the shows with a large share of children in the audience are not necessarily the shows that have the largest number of children watching. And the relationship between child audience share and child audience size, or the number of children watching, may vary across the different sources of programming. This section examines these issues.

We group shows by size according to whether they are watched by fewer than 1 percent of children, between 1 and 3 percent of children, or more than 3 percent of children. We find that, in our data, there are no shows watched by more than 10 percent of children and few (less than 1 percent) watched by more than 5 percent of children. In contrast, 86 percent of shows are watched by fewer than 0.2 percent of children and 96 percent are watched by fewer than 1 percent of children. As indicated in Table 3.7, about half of children's ad exposure comes from shows with fewer than 1 percent of children watching and less than 20 percent of exposure comes from shows watched by more than 3 percent of children.

Table 3.7 presents the distribution of ad exposure for ads by child audience size, as measured by Gross Rating Points (GRPs), and child audience share for our data. The top panel illustrates this distribution for all ads. Each cell in the central box represents the percentage of ad exposure that comes from shows with a given size and share combination. We see that 13.4 percent of all child ad exposures come from programs for which at least 50 percent of the audience is children and which are seen by more than 3 percent of the child population. In contrast, only 3.2 percent of the ads are seen on programs with a small share of children in the audience but more than three percent of children watching. There is a distinct pattern observable in this table — 41.2 percent of exposure comes from shows with a small children's share and a small number of children watching (GRP less than one), while 31.3 percent comes from shows with a high children's share, at least 50 percent, and with at least 1 percent of children watching.[34]

Table 3.7. Percent of Ad Exposure By Audience Size (GRP) and Audience Share

Children ages 211

All ads   25,629 ads

		Share		
GRP		0-20	20-50	≥ 50	Total
0.0 –	1.0	41.2	5.3	2.5	49.1
1.0 –	3.0	8.6	5.9	17.9	32.4
≥ 3.0		3.2	1.9	13.4	18.5
Total		53.0	13.1	33.8	100.0

Ads on Cable   61.4% exposure

	Share			
GRP	0-20	20-50	≥ 50	Total
0.0 – 1.0	35.5	6.1	3.9	45.5
1.0 – 3.0	0.3	5.2	28.7	34.2
≥ 3.0	0.0	0.0	20.3	20.3
Total	35.8	11.3	52.9	100.0

Ads on Broadcast   38.6% exposure

	Share			
GRP	0-20	20-50	≥ 50	Total
0.0 – 1.0	50.4	4.2	0.3	54.9
1.0 – 3.0	21.8	7.0	0.9	29.6
≥ 3.0	8.3	4.9	2.3	15.5
Total	80.4	16.1	3.5	100.0

Source: Staff analysis of copyrighted Nielsen Media Research/Nielsen Monitor–Plus data; four weeks projected annually.

The second panel summarizes the data on cable ads. We see that the pattern of cable ads is similar to that for all national ads. This is to be expected since children get 61.4 percent of their ad exposure from cable television. However, on cable, 49 percent of exposure comes from shows with a high children's share, at least 50 percent, and at least one percent of the child population watching. Also, all the cable shows with a viewership greater than 3 percent of the child population also have a children's audience share greater than 50 percent. The bulk of children's remaining ad exposure from cable channels, 35.5 percent, comes from shows with fewer children in the audience and with a children's audience share of less than 20 percent.

Table 3.8. Percent of Food Ad Exposure By Audience Size (GRP) and Audience Share

Children ages 211

All ads   5,538 ads

GRP	Share 020	2050	> 50	Total
0.01.0	27.1	4.7	3.0	34.8
1.03.0	7.0	6.6	25.4	39.0
>3.0	2.5	1.8	22.0	26.3
Total	36.5	13.0	50.4	100.0

Ads on cable   72.0% exposure

GRP	Share 0–20	20–50	> 50	Total
0.0 – 1.0	21.6	4.9	4.1	30.6
1.0 – 3.0	0.2	4.8	34.9	39.9
>3.0	0.0	0.0	29.4	29.4
Total	21.8	9.8	68.4	100.0

Ads on broadcast   28.0% exposure

GRP	Share 0–20	20–50	> 50	Total
0.0 – 1.0	41.1	4.1	0.3	45.5
1.03.0	24.3	11.1	1.0	36.4
>3.0	8.8	6.3	3.0	18.1
Total	74.3	21.5	4.2	100.0

Source: Staff analysis of copyrighted Nielsen Media Research/Nielsen Monitor–Plus data; four weeks projected annually.

The third panel summarizes the data on broadcast ads. Broadcast advertising accounts for 38.6 percent of children's exposure to ads. This panel indicates that very few broadcast shows have a high children's audience share; these shows provide 3.5 percent of children's broadcast ad exposure. Those broadcast shows with children's audience share of less than 20 percent account for 80.4 percent of children's exposure to broadcast advertising.

Thus, this evidence indicates that any advertising restrictions based on children's share of a show's audience would primarily affect cable programming; the vast majority of advertising exposure on broadcast programming is from shows with a child audience share of less than 20 percent.

Food Advertising

Table 3.8 presents the comparable child audience distribution data as Table 3.7, but restricted to food advertising. The audience pattern is similar to the overall distribution, with children's food ad exposure somewhat more concentrated on cable programming and on children's programming on cable networks.

In this case we find that, for all food ads, 47.4 percent of children's exposure comes from programming with a high children's share and with a children's audience of at least one percent of the child population. A much smaller fraction of their food ad exposure, 27.2 percent, comes from shows with a low children's share and a small children's audience. Overall, children's exposure to food ads is more concentrated in children's programming than exposure to ads for other products; 50.4 percent of exposure to food ads comes from shows with a children's share of at least 50 percent, compared to 33.8 percent of exposure to ads for all products.

We also see that children's exposure to food ads is somewhat more concentrated on cable programming — 72.0 percent of children's food ad exposure comes from cable, compared to 61.4 of all ad exposure. On cable programming 68.4 percent of food ad exposure comes from shows with a children's share of at least 50 percent, compared to 52.9 percent of exposure to ads for all products. While 35.5 percent of cable ads are seen on programs with an audience that has a small child share (less than 20 percent) and size (less than 1 percent of all children), only 21.6 percent of the cable food ad exposures occur on these programs.

Thus, as with children's exposure to advertising generally, any restrictions on food advertising based on children's audience share would primarily affect cable programming.

Table 3.9. Annual Exposure to TV Advertising

Younger children ages 2–5, older children ages 6–11, and children ages 2–11

Category	2–5		6–11		2–11	
	Ads	%	Ads	%	Ads	%
Cereal	1,031	4.1	968	3.7	993	3.9
Desserts and Sweets	857	3.4	925	3.5	898	3.5
Restaurants and Fast Food	1,252	5.0	1,442	5.5	1,367	5.3
Snacks	499	2.0	484	1.9	490	1.9
Dairy Products	370	1.5	342	1.3	353	1.4
Sweetened Drinks	388	1.6	457	1.8	430	1.7
Prepared Entrees	218	0.9	224	0.9	222	0.9
Other Food	776	3.1	793	3.0	786	3.1
All Food Products	**5,390**	**21.6**	**5,635**	**21.6**	**5,538**	**21.6**
Games, Toys and Hobbies	2,092	8.4	1,791	6.9	1,909	7.5
Screen / Audio Entertainment	1,853	7.4	2,113	8.1	2,010	7.8
Sports and Exercise	21	0.1	25	0.1	24	0.1
Promos and PSAs	7,270	29.2	7,328	28.1	7,305	28.5
Other Nonfood	8,314	33.3	9,186	35.2	8,842	34.5
All Nonfood Products	**19,549**	**78.4**	**20,443**	**78.4**	**20,091**	**78.4**
Total	**24,939**		**26,079**		**25,629**	

Source: Staff analysis of copyrighted Nielsen Media Research/Nielsen Monitor–Plus data; four weeks projected annually.

3.6. Younger Children

Some research points to particular effects of advertising on younger children who may not comprehend the intent of advertisers. The position of the American Academy of Pediatrics is that advertising directed to young children is inherently deceptive and exploits children younger than eight (Shifrin 2005). While our evidence does not address young children's ability to understand the selling intent of advertising, we can provide some data on whether the mix of product advertising seen by younger children is different from that of older children in the larger group analyzed in the chapter so far. Our data allow us to look at the standard industry age groups 25, 611, and 211.

Children ages 2–5 see, on average, 5,390 food ads per year and 19,549 ads for other products — a total of 24,939 ads per year. The first two columns of Table 3.9 show younger children's average annual ad exposure in each product category along with the percentage contribution of that category to total ad exposure. Younger children's television ad exposure is very similar to that of children ages 6–11, shown in the second set of columns. The younger children see 1,140 fewer ads per year than 6–11 year olds, on average, primarily because they are watching slightly less television than older children. However, the mix of products they view in ads is strikingly similar to that viewed by children 6–11. The largest differences are in Games, Toys and Hobbies which contribute 1.5 percentage points more to younger children's exposure and Other Nonfood which contributes 1.9 percentage points less to their exposure. Within the food categories, the largest differences are that younger children see more Cereal ads and fewer ads for Restaurants and Fast Food, but both differences are smaller than one percentage point.

Table 3.10. Annual Exposure to TV Advertising By Younger Children's Share of Audience

Younger children ages 2–5

Category	All ads		Share ≥ 20%		Share ≥ 50%	
	Ads	%	Ads	%	Ads	%
Cereal	1,031	4.1	770	8.6	79	8.3
Desserts and Sweets	857	3.4	477	5.3	6	0.7
Restaurants and Fast Food	252	5.0	456	5.1	50	5.2
Snacks	499	2.0	331	3.7	18	1.9
Dairy Products	370	1.5	251	2.8	28	2.9
Sweetened Drinks	388	1.6	147	1.6	0	0.0
Prepared Entrees	218	0.9	106	1.2	5	0.6
Other Food	776	3.1	226	2.5	41	4.2
All Food Products	**5,390**	**21.6**	**2,764**	**30.8**	**227**	**23.8**
Games, Toys and Hobbies	092	8.4	1, 710	19.0	217	22.8
Screen / Audio Entertainment	1, 853	7.4	846	9.4	38	4.0
Sports and Exercise	21	0.1	11	0.1	0	0.0
Promos and PSAs	7, 270	29.2	2, 575	28.7	214	22.4
Other Nonfood	8, 314	33.3	1, 078	12.0	258	27.0
All Nonfood Products	**19, 549**	**78.4**	**6, 220**	**69.2**	**727**	**76.2**
Total	**24,939**		**8,985**		**954**	

Source: Staff analysis of copyrighted Nielsen Media Research/Nielsen Monitor–Plus data; four weeks projected annually.

Table 3.11. Percent of Ad Exposure by Audience Size (GRP) and Audience Share

Younger children ages 25

All ads		Share		24,939 ads	
GRP	020	2050	> 50	Total	
0.0	1.0	45.3	3.3	0.1	48.6
1.0	3.0	15.0	13.8	0.0	28.8
>3.0		3.8	15.1	3.7	22.6
Total		64.0	32.2	3.8	100.0

Ads on cable		Share		64.2% exposure
GRP	0–20	20–50	> 50	Total
0.0 – 1.0	38.2	4.9	0.1	43.2
1.0 – 3.0	7.3	20.9	0.0	28.2
>3.0	0.3	22.6	5.7	28.6
Total	45.8	48.4	5.8	100.0

Ads on broadcast		Share		35.8% exposure
GRP	0–20	20–50	> 50	Total
0.0 – 1.0	57.8	0.5	0.0	58.3
1.03.0	28.7	1.1	0.1	29.8
>3.0	10.0	1.7	0.2	11.9
Total	96.5	3.2	0.3	100.0

Source: Staff analysis of copyrighted Nielsen Media Research/Nielsen Monitor–Plus data; four weeks projected annually.

Unlike children 211, younger children get only a small percentage of their television ad exposure from shows in which they make up at least a 50 percent share of the audience.[35] Table 3.10 presents the number of ads and percent of ad exposure from shows categorized by their share of children 2–5 years of age. The table shows that younger children get only 4.2 percent of their food ad exposure, and 3.8 percent of total exposure, on shows in which they are at least half of the audience. Younger children get 51.3 percent of their food ad exposure on shows in which they make up at least 20 percent of the audience; they get 36.0 percent of total ad exposure from those shows.

Table 3.11 presents the distribution of the audience of younger children (2–5) by young child audience size and audience share. Younger children get 64.0 percent of their exposure to ads from shows with a 2–5 audience share less than 20 percent. Nearly half their ad exposure is on shows with a small 2–5 audience size, that is, less than one percent of the 25 population. Younger children get 64.2 percent of their annual advertising exposure from cable programming, compared to 61.4 percent for children 2–11. They get 38.6 percent of their exposure from broadcast programming. But virtually all of that broadcast exposure (96.5 percent) is from shows in which younger children make up less than 20 percent of the audience.

Taken together, this evidence indicates that any restrictions on advertising based on audience share for younger children (25) would affect only cable programming. And if restricted to programs with more than a 50 percent share of younger children, these restrictions would affect few programs and few of the ads that these children see.

3.7. Teenagers and Adults

Table 3.12 presents estimated annual ad exposure for teenagers and adults, as well as children, to allow us to compare ad exposures across the three age groups.

Teenagers (those ages 12–17) see, on average, 31,188 ads per year — 5,512 food ads and 25,677 ads for other goods. Food ads constitute 17.7 percent of all the ads teens saw in 2004, a somewhat smaller proportion than that for children. The largest categories of food ads viewed are Restaurants and Fast Food (5.9 percent of all ad exposure), Desserts and Sweets (2.6 percent), and Sweetened Drinks (1.9 percent).

The largest nonfood categories are Promos and PSAs (25.7 percent of all advertising exposure) and Screen/Audio Entertainment (8.4 percent). Games, Toys and Hobbies contribute only 2.5 percent to teenagers' ad exposure.

Adults, on average, see 52,469 ads per year — 7,212 food ads and 45,257 ads for other products. Food ads constitute 13.7 percent of all the ads adults saw in 2004. The only sizeable food category in adults' ad exposure is Restaurants and Fast Food, at 4.9 percent. Promos and PSAs make up 24.1 percent of their overall exposure to advertising.

Table 3.12. Annual Exposure to TV Advertising

Children ages 2–11, teens ages 12–17 and adults ages 18 and over

Category	Children		Teens		Adults	
	Ads	%	Ads	%	Ads	%
Cereal	993	3.9	492	1.6	477	0.9
Desserts and Sweets	898	3.5	806	2.6	754	1.4
Restaurants and Fast Food	1,367	5.3	1,836	5.9	2,546	4.9
Snacks	490	1.9	332	1.1	356	0.7
Dairy Products	353	1.4	260	0.8	338	0.6
Sweetened Drinks	430	1.7	584	1.9	479	0.9
Prepared Entrees	222	0.9	180	0.6	323	0.6
Other Food	786	3.1	1,021	3.3	1,939	3.7
All Food Products	**5,538**	**21.6**	**5,512**	**17.7**	**7,212**	**13.7**
Games, Toys and Hobbies	909	7.5	778	2.5	414	0.8
Screen / Audio Entertainment	010	7.8	2, 633	8.4	2, 323	4.4
Sports and Exercise	24	0.1	24	0.1	47	0.1
Promos and PSAs	305	28.5	8, 007	25.7	12, 627	24.1
Other Nonfood	842	34.5	14, 235	45.6	29, 846	56.9
All Nonfood Products	**20, 091**	**78.4**	**25, 677**	**82.3**	**45, 257**	**86.3**
Total	**25,629**		**31,188**		**52,469**	

Source: Staff analysis of copyrighted Nielsen Media Research/Nielsen Monitor–Plus data;
    four weeks projected annually.

The Other Nonfood category contributes the most to overall advertising exposure for all age groups. It is 34.5 percent of children's overall exposure, 45.6 percent of teenager's overall exposure, and 56.9 percent of adults overall advertising exposure. Services and products in Other Nonfood include clothing and accessories, prescription and OTC drugs, professional services, schools and camps, utilities, communication services, financial services, insurance, realtors, books, and personal hygiene products.[36]

The overall differences in total advertising exposures across these groups primarily reflect differences in television viewing time. Estimates based on our Nielsen data indicate that adults watch nearly twice as much commercially-sponsored television as children (4 hours 10 minutes versus 2 hours 17 minutes, or 82 percent more than children), and teenagers watch 10 percent more than children. The differences in ad exposure are, to a lesser degree, a result of the different number of ads per hour viewed by the different age groups. Children see about 31 ads per hour, teenagers see about 34 ads per hour, and adults see about

35 ads per hour. Advertising exposures for adults and teenagers, compared to children, are only slightly larger than viewing differences would suggest; the remaining difference is due to adults and teenagers viewing more ads per hour.

4. TELEVISION ADVERTISING IN 1977

Two studies were done in 1978 for the FTC Children's Advertising Rulemaking.[37] Both examined the products featured in television advertising seen by children and others. Abel (1978) focused on a subset of nationally aired ads, and Beales (1978) focused on locally generated spot ads. These studies were completed before children's obesity and overweight began rising. Therefore, they provide a good baseline as we attempt to assess whether changes in television advertising may have contributed to the increase in overweight and obesity in children.

Table 4.1 details the data analyzed by each of the reports. Abel did not analyze the national ads aired on all network shows. His analysis was restricted to shows with at least a 20 percent child audience share or at least 3.5 million child viewers. He also analyzed the subsets with at least a 30 percent child audience share, a 50 percent audience share, a 5 million child audience size, and an 8 million child audience size. The local spot ads in the Beales' study could not be analyzed at the show level, because different shows were being aired in different locations. Therefore, Beales analyzed shows based on dayparts — the time of day and day of the week the ads were seen. (Table 4.5 gives the definitions of these dayparts.) Beales analyzed ads aired on all dayparts, as well as three subsets of those dayparts — those with at least a 20 percent child audience share, a 30 percent audience share, and a 50 percent audience share.

4.1. Abel's Study of National Advertising

Abel's research examined children's exposure to national network television advertising and compared it to overall audience exposure. Specifically, he considers two questions: "(1) to what products and product categories are children exposed in network advertising? and (2) what percentage of the total amount of network advertising of these products is contained in programs that children watch?" (Abel 1978, pp. 5). Abel used network audience data from Arbitron and advertising data from Broadcast Advertisers Reports.[38] The data were from

February, May, and November 1977. The analysis is focused on two groups of television programs: those with the largest share of children in the audience, and those with the largest numbers of children in the audience. Specifically, Abel analyzed advertising on the 50 shows with the largest children's audience share for each of the three months in his data, along with advertising on the 50 shows with the largest number of children in the audience for each of the three months. His analysis of exposure to advertising — combining information on ads aired with data on the audience ratings — was further restricted to those shows with at least a 20 percent child audience share or at least 3.5 million children in the audience.

4.1.1. Overview of National Network Television Landscape in the Late 1970s

The three network shows with the largest share of children in the audience for February and May were "Jabberjaw," "Captain Kangaroo," and "Tom-Jerry-Mumbly Show;" children made up between 72 and 76 percent of their audiences. In November, the three shows with the largest children's audience share were "All New Superfriends Hour," "Captain Kangaroo," and "C B Bears;" children made up between 69 and 71 percent of their audiences. Children made up between 15 and 19 percent of the audience for shows at the bottom of the list of the 50 shows with the highest children's audience share. Examples of shows in this range include "Gong Show," "The Price is Right," "Good Times," and "Family Feud." Overall, in 1977 there were fewer than 25 shows with a child audience share greater than 50 percent.

Table 4.1. Coverage of the Abel and Beales Reports

	Abel	Beales
Source of advertising	Network	Non-network
Unit of analysis	Shows	Dayparts
Data coverage		
All programming	Yes	
Child share ≥ 20%	Yes	Yes
Child share ≥ 30%	Yes	Yes
Child share ≥ 50%	Yes	Yes
Child audience ≥ 3.5 million	Yes	
Child audience ≥ 5 million	Yes	
Child audience ≥ 8 million	Yes	

Source: Abel (1978); Beales (1978).
Note: Child refers to a child ages 2–11.

The two shows with the largest number of children in the audience for all three months were "Happy Days" and "Laverne and Shirley." "Happy Days" had between 10 and 16 million children in the audience in these three months. Shows with the fiftieth largest children's audience ("Charlie's Angels," "Tom-Jerry-Mumbly Show," and "Superwitch") had between 2 and 3 million children in the audience, audiences comparable in size to the leading children's shows by audience share. The population aged 2 through 11 was approximately 33.6 million in early 1977 in America, so the highest rated shows by child audience size were being watched by close to half of all children in some months, but these shows did not have high child audience shares. Thus, the shows that reached most children in 1977 were not children's shows.

4.1.2 Analysis of Products Advertised

Abel analyzed exposure to advertising in 26 product categories.[39] Table 4.2 lists those categories. As before, we simplify by aggregating some of his detailed categories into fewer categories.

In analyzing the programs with the largest children's audience share, Abel separately looked at programs with more than 20 percent, 30 percent, and 50 percent children in the audience.[40,41] In the analysis of programs with the largest number of children viewers, he separately looked at shows with more than 3.5 million, 5 million, and 8 million children in the audience.[42] These numbers of viewers correspond to approximately 10.7 percent, 15.2 percent, and 24.4 percent of the U.S. population of children in 1977.

Table 4.3 summarizes Abel's findings regarding children's exposure to national advertising on programs in which children make up a significant share of the audience. Consider advertising on programs for which at least 50 percent of the audience was children. Nearly 62 percent of the ads were for food or beverages and more than half of those, 32 percent of the total, were for cereals. In the nonfood arena, advertising for Games, Toys and Hobbies constitutes 90 percent of the ads (34.3 out of 38.1 percentage points). The three categories of Cereal, Desserts and Sweets, and Games, Toys and Hobbies constitute 83 percent of all ads children saw on these shows. Thus, on these shows with child audience shares of at least 50 percent national advertising was very highly concentrated to these "big three" categories, as reported by other studies of the time in the literature, using different approaches. On shows with 20 percent or more of children in the audience, these three categories are still important, but their share has dropped to 58 percent of ads.

Table 4.2. Composition of Summary Categories in 1977
Categories Abel's Detailed Categories

Categories	Abel's Detailed Categories
Cereal	Regular Cereal
	Highly Sugared Cereal
Desserts and Sweets	Candy
	Desserts and Dessert Ingredients
	Cakes, Pies and Pastries
	Regular Gum
	Cookies
	Ice Cream
Snacks	Appetizers, Snacks and Nuts
	Crackers
Sweetened Drinks	Regular Carbonated Beverages
	Non-carbonated Beverages
Restaurants and Fast Food	Restaurants and Drive-ins
Other Food Products	Beer, Wine and Mixers
	Diet Carbonated Beverages
	Fruit Juices
	Sugarless Gum
	Canned Fruit
	Raisins
	Fresh Fruit
	Other Food and Beverages
Games, Toys and Hobbies	Games, Toys and Hobbies
Bicycles	Bicycles
Other Nonfood Prodcuts	Dental Supplies
	Footwear
	Other Nonfood Advertising

Note: Beales (1978) used the same categories as Abel (1978).

For programs with 20 percent or more children in the audience, food's share of children's advertising exposure dropped to around 58 percent, but this is only a four percentage point drop from the 50 percent share shows. Advertising for Other Food and Beverages increased, primarily drawing share away from Cereal and Desserts and Sweets, but Food is a major portion of national advertising on all these show types in 1977.

**Table 4.3. Annual Exposure to National Advertising in 1977
by Audience Share**

Children ages 2–11, national advertising

Category	Share ≥ 20%		Share ≥ 30%		Share ≥ 50%	
	Ads	%	Ads	%	Ads	%
Cereal	595	21.8	548	29.7	513	32.0
Desserts and Sweets	373	13.7	302	16.3	271	16.9
Restaurants and Fast Food	113	4.1	58	3.1	52	3.3
Snacks	35	1.3	20	1.1	13	0.8
Sweetened Drinks	62	2.3	33	1.8	25	1.6
Other Food	401	14.7	145	7.8	118	7.4
All Food Products	**1,579**	**57.7**	**1,105**	**59.9**	**993**	**61.9**
Games, Toys and Hobbies	610	22.3	593	32.1	551	34.3
Sports and Exercise	0	0.0	0	0.0	8	0.5
Other Nonfood	546	20.0	148	8.0	52	3.3
All Nonfood Products	**1, 156**	**42.3**	**741**	**40.1**	**611**	**38.1**
Total	**2,735**		**1,846**		**1,604**	

Source: Abel (1978, Tables XVI, XVII and XVIII).

Note: Share refers to the average child share of the audience for each show. Abel (1978) did not report exposure to advertising on all shows.

The next table provides advertising exposure based on the numbers of children watching particular shows. Table 4.4 gives children's exposure to national advertising on shows with at least 3.5 million children viewers, 5 million children viewers, and 8 million viewing. Thus, on the shows with large child audiences, food advertising is still substantial, but no longer the majority of the ads seen. Also the big three categories (Cereal, Games, Toys and Hobbies, and Desserts and Sweets) are no longer dominant, constituting only 31 percent of ads seen for shows with more than 3.5 million children in the audience, and only 21 percent of ads for shows with more than eight million children. Thus, the Abel study shows that the standard finding in the literature — that children's advertising was highly concentrated to the big three categories — is dependent on measuring shows where children are a large share of the audience, but in 1977 these were not shows which were seen by the largest numbers of children.

**Table 4.4. Annual Exposure to National Advertising in 1977
by Audience Size**

Children ages 2–11, national advertising

Category	Size ≥ 3.5 million		Size ≥ 5 million		Share ≥ 8 million	
	Ads	%	Ads	%	Ads	%
Cereal	303	10.5	189	9.1	78	6.4
Desserts and Sweets	273	9.5	166	8.0	50	4.2
Restaurants and Fast Food	116	4.0	84	4.0	53	4.4
Snacks	127	4.4	113	5.4	8	0.7
Sweetened Drinks	53	1.8	37	1.8	17	1.4
Other Food	483	16.8	373	17.9	271	22.4
All Food Products	**1, 355**	**47.1**	**961**	**46.1**	**477**	**39.5**
Games, Toys and Hobbies	313	10.9	179	8.6	127	10.6
Sports and Exercise	0	0.0	0	0.0	0	0.0
Other Nonfood	1, 209	42.0	945	45.3	602	49.9
All Nonfood Products	**1, 522**	**52.9**	**1, 124**	**53.9**	**730**	**60.5**
Total	**2,877**		**2,086**		**1,207**	

Source: Abel (1978, Tables XIX, XX and XI).
Note: Audience size refers to the average number of child viewers for each show. Abel (1978) did not report exposure to advertising on all shows.

4.2. Beales' Study of Spot Ads

Beales' 1978 research examined the patterns of children's and adults' exposure to spot television advertising.[43] Spot television is defined as non-network advertising that local network affiliates and independent stations carry for local, regional or national advertisers (Abel 1978). Advertising data were obtained from Broadcast Advertiser's Reports, Inc., and covered approximately 267 television stations located in 75 of the largest US television markets. Each station was monitored for one week in each of four months — February, May, July, and November of 1977. These data were matched with audience data from Arbitron Television Daypart Audience Summary to capture exposure to advertising. Data were accumulated separately for each of 17 dayparts. Dayparts are defined as a specified period of time, on a specified day (or days) of the week, on a specified station. Table 4.5 lists these dayparts. This is the unit of analysis for this research, which is similar to the concept of a program, though a daypart typically contains more than one program and is thus not directly comparable to Abel's program analysis or our 2004 analysis.[44]

The Beales advertising data were categorized into the same 26 product categories used by Abel (see Table 4.2). In analyzing exposure to advertising, Beales looked at the distribution of advertising across all product classes, for all dayparts, and those dayparts with 20 percent, 30 percent and 50 percent children in the audience. Table 4.6 shows the estimated annual exposure to local ads by category from all dayparts (all programming), and dayparts for which children make up at least 20 percent, 30 percent, and 50 percent of the audience. This table shows that toy advertising dominates on local advertising. Children are exposed to about three times as much advertising for Games, Toys and Hobbies as for Cereal, the largest category of food advertising exposure. Over all dayparts, food advertising makes up 26 percent of all children's advertising exposure on local ads. When restricted to dayparts where at least 50 percent of the audience is children, food advertising is nearly 27 percent of all local advertising seen by children; in these shows, 29 percent of ad exposure is from toy advertising.

Table 4.5. Dayparts Used in Beales' Analysis

	Eastern & Pacific		Central & Mountain	
Monday – Friday	7:00 am	– 9:00 am	7:00 am	– 9:00 am
	9:00 am	– Noon	9:00 am	– Noon
	Noon	– 4:30 pm	Noon	– 3:30 pm
	4:30 pm	– 6:00 pm	3:30 pm	– 5:00 pm
	6:00 pm	– 7:30 pm	5:00 pm	– 6:30 pm
	7:30 pm	– 8:00 pm	6:30 pm	– 7:00 pm
	11:00 pm	– 11:30 pm	10:00 pm	– 10:30 pm
	11:30 pm	– 1:00 am	10:30 pm	– Midnight
Saturday	8:30 am	– 1:00 pm	8:30 am	– 1:00 pm
Saturday & Sunday	1:00 pm	– 5:00 pm	1:00 pm	– 4:00 pm
Sunday – Saturday	8:00 pm	– 11:00 pm	7:00 pm	– 10:00 pm

Source: Beales (1978, Table A2).

The share of food ad exposures is fairly steady between 25 and 27 percent as the fraction of children in the audience increases. Cereal ads contribute an increasing portion of advertising exposure as the share of children in the audience increases — from four percent in all programming to 10 percent in dayparts with 50 percent or more children. Dessert and Sweets ads increase slightly in prevalence as the share of children grows, as do ads for Restaurants and Fast Food. Ads for Sweetened Drinks and Other Food decline in prevalence as the share of children increases. Ads for Games, Toys and Hobbies increase more substantially as children's share of audience increases — these are 12 percent of exposure on all programming and 29 percent of exposure in dayparts in which children have at least a 50 percent share.

Food advertising was a far smaller portion of children's exposure from local advertising in 1977 than from national advertising on shows with a children's share of at least 20 percent. However, ads for Restaurants and Fast Food made up a slightly larger fraction of exposure to spot ads, 5.6 percent, than of exposure to national network ads on these shows, 5.2 percent. Toy advertising was also a much more substantial part of local advertising than in national advertising in 1977.

Table 4.6. Annual Exposure to Local Advertising in 1977 by Daypart Audience Share

Children ages 2–11, local advertising

Category	All dayparts		Share ≥ 20%		Share ≥ 30%		Share ≥ 50%	
	Ads	%	Ads	%	Ads	%	Ads	%
Cereal	469	4.2	433	6.3	405	7.4	282	10.3
Desserts and Sweets	546	4.9	420	6.1	346	6.4	176	6.4
Restaurants and Fast Food	632	5.6	379	5.5	305	5.6	169	6.1
Snacks	38	0.3	14	0.2	8	0.1	2	0.1
Sweetened Drinks	273	2.4	146	2.1	101	1.9	36	1.3
Other Food	984	8.8	380	5.5	241	4.4	70	2.5
All Food Products	**2,941**	**26.3**	**1,774**	**25.7**	**1,406**	**25.8**	**735**	**26.7**
Games, Toys and Hobbies	1,359	12.1	1,305	18.9	1,199	22.0	793	28.8
Sports and Exercise	30	0.3	28	0.4	25	0.5	12	0.4
Other Nonfood	6,864	61.3	3,793	55.0	2,813	51.7	1,211	44.0
All Nonfood Products	**8,253**	**73.7**	**5,125**	**74.3**	**4,037**	**74.2**	**2,015**	**73.3**
Total	**11,194**		**6,899**		**5,443**		**2,751**	

Source: Beales (1978, Tables 1, B-3, B-6 and B-9).
Note: Columns reflect exposure to advertising when children constitute at least 20%, 30%, and 50% of the average audience for a daypart.

5. WHAT CAN WE SAY ABOUT 1977 AND 2004?

One of our goals in this study is to examine how children's exposure to television advertising has changed from 1977 to 2004. We use Abel (1978), Beales (1978), and an NSF study, Adler et al. (1977), to assess how children's exposure has changed. Children's exposure to television advertising rose slightly from 1977 to 2004, due to increased exposure to Promos. Children's exposure to food advertising almost certainly declined, in our estimate by about 9 percent.

5.1. Children's Overall Ad Exposure: 1977 and 2004

We cannot compute children's overall exposure to television advertising directly from Abel (1978) and Beales (1978) because Abel did not analyze children's exposure to advertising on all network shows. Instead, we turn to other publicly available information for children's exposure to advertising in 1977.

A 1977 National Science Foundation study headed by Richard Adler examined children's exposure to television advertising from all programming. The study estimated that children ages 2–11 saw, on average, 21,904 ads per year, 19,714 of which were paid ads (Adler et al. 1977). Throughout this section, we use the Adler et al. (1977) estimate for children's overall exposure to advertising in 1977.[45]

Table 5.1 presents our 2004 estimates, as well as those based on the Adler study. Note that, in 2004, children, ages 2–11, are estimated to have seen 18,324 paid ads — 7 percent fewer paid ads than in the late 1970s. However, the large increase in Promos and PSAs seen by children led to a 17 percent increase in overall ad exposure; in 2004, children, on average, saw 25,629 ads, up from 21,904 in 1977. Two countervailing factors contributed to these changes. First, children, on average, watched fewer hours of TV per day in 2004 than in 1977; they watched even fewer hours of ad-supported TV. Second, the number of ads aired per hour increased from 19 in 1977 to 30 in 2004 (Adler et al. 1977).

The table also provides data on exposure to minutes of television advertising, in addition to numbers of ads. Because the average length of television ads has declined since 1977 (from approximately 30 seconds to 25 seconds), children's exposure to minutes of advertising has declined, both for paid ads and for all advertising.[46] Minutes of paid ad exposure for children declined from 9,857 in 1977 to 7,987 in 2004. Minutes of overall ad exposure fell from 10,952 to 10,717, a smaller percentage decline than the exposure to paid ads, again due to the marked increase in minutes of Promos and PSAs.

The table also provides analogous information for children 25 and 611. The patterns are similar to those for children 2–11, except that exposure to paid ads fell more for the 2–5 year-olds and exposure to overall ads grew less for these younger children.

Table 5.1. Estimated TV Advertising Viewed by Children: 1977 and 2004

Type of ad	Ads viewed			Ad minutes viewed		
	1977	2004	% change	1977	2004	% change
Children ages 2–11	21,904	25,629	17%	10,952	10,717	-2%
Paid advertisements	19,714	18,324	-7%	9,857	7,987	-19%
Promos[a] and PSAs[b]	2,190	7,305	234%	1,095	2,730	149%
Younger children ages 2–5	22,571	24,939	10%	11,376	10,425	-8%
Paid advertisements	20,476	17,669	-14%	10,238	7,678	-25%
Promos[a] and PSAs[b]	2,275	7,270	220%	1,138	2,747	141%
Older children ages 6–11	21,373	26,079	22%	10,687	10,908	2%
Paid advertisements	19,236	18,750	-3%	9,618	8,189	-15%
Promos[a] and PSAs[b]	2,137	7,328	243%	1,069	2,719	154%

Source: Staff estimates based on Adler et al. (1977) for 1977. Staff analysis of copyrighted Nielsen Media Research/Nielsen Monitor–Plus data; four weeks projected annually for 2004.

Note: [a]Promotional advertisements for an outlet's own or affiliated shows. [b]Public Service Announcements.

5.2. Exposure to Food Advertising: 1977 and 2004

The two reports by Abel and Beales are, to date, the most comprehensive analyses of children's exposure to television advertising. Since they look at children's ad exposure in 1977 prior to the rise in children's obesity rates, these reports provide a baseline against which to compare recent exposure to television advertising. However, some limitations should be noted in comparing the 1977 and 2004 results.

First, the two 1977 reports are not directly comparable to each other. Abel had ratings data and advertisement descriptions at the TV program level. Because Beales was examining local spot ads, and programming varies by locality, his units of observation were dayparts. Therefore, Beales' dayparts with a particular child audience share are not directly comparable to Abel's shows with such a share. Of course, it would be legitimate to compare, and combine, children's exposure on all shows and all dayparts. This brings us to the second limitation.

Abel did not analyze exposure to advertising on all network shows, only those for which children were at least 20 percent of the audience.[47] Thus, we do not have a direct measure of the pattern of children's overall exposure to ads in the various product categories; the ads from network shows with less than 20 percent child audience share are missing. Despite these limitations, together with other information from the period including Adler et al. (1977) — much can be learned from the comparisons that can be made.

To assess whether children are seeing more or less food advertising in 2004 compared to 1977, we begin by using the Adler et al. (1977) estimate of children's overall exposure to advertising to obtain an estimate of the amount of network advertising exposure that is missing from Abel's analysis. Adler et al. (1977) estimated that children saw 21,904 ads, 2,190 (10 percent of the total) of which were Promos and PSAs. Recall that neither Abel nor Beales had estimates of exposure to Promos or PSAs. Table 5.2 summarizes the data we have from various studies under the assumption that the percentage of Promos and PSAs was distributed evenly across the types of programming,[48] and shows that an estimated 6,427 ad exposures must have come from the missing network programs with a child audience share of less than 20 percent.[49]

We do not know the composition of the ads in the missing data. However, by using other information from 1977, we can establish that children's food advertising exposure has almost certainly declined overall, and we can gauge the approximate size of the decrease.

We look at the issue in two ways. Table 5.3 summarizes food advertising as a percent of all advertising on shows with various child audience shares in 1977 and 2004. In both years, the share of food advertising falls somewhat for network and non-network programming as the programming becomes more general (that is, as child audience share falls). For national network ads in 2004, children's food ad exposure on all shows was 22.6 percent, compared to 32.6 percent on shows with a 50 percent child share; thus the percentage of food ads on all shows was 30.7 percent less than that on the 50 percent share shows.[50] If the reduction for all shows compared to children's shows was of a similar magnitude in 1977, the percentage of food ads on all national shows in 1977 would be approximately 42.9 percent.[51]

**Table 5.2. Children's Exposure Estimates From Available Studies:
1977 and 2004**

	Paid Advertising			Promos &	
	Food	Nonfood	Total	PSAs	Total
1977					
Adler			19,714	2,190	21,904
Abel	1,579	1,156	2,735	304[b]	3,039[a]
Beales	2,941	8,253	11,194	1,244[b]	12,438[a]
Missing	1, 564[d]	4, 221[d]	5, 785	643[b]	6, 427[c]
2004					
FTC	5,538	12,786	18,324	7,305	25,629

Source: Staff estimates based on Abel (1978), Beales (1978), and Adler et al. (1977) for 1977. Staff analysis of copyrighted Nielsen Media Research/Nielsen Monitor–Plus data; four weeks projected annually for 2004.

Note: [a]Estimated assuming Promos and PSAs constitute 10 percent of advertising. [b]Estimated assuming Promos and PSAs constitute 10 percent of advertising. [c]Total advertising from Adler less local advertising from Beales and national advertising on shows with child audience share at least 20% from Abel. [d]Estimated assuming that national food advertising constitutes 33.2 percent of all national advertising, as discussed below.

**Table 5.3. Children's Exposure to Food Ads As a Percent of All Exposure by
Show Type: 1977 and 2004**

	All Shows	20%+ Share	50%+ Share
1977			
Network Ads (Abel)[a]		57.7	61.9
Non-network Ads (Beales)[b]	26.3	25.7	26.7
2004			
Network Ads[a]	22.6	30.2	32.6
Non-network Ads[b]	16.8	19.5	20.1

Source: Staff estimates based on Abel (1978, Tables XVI, XVII and XVIII) and Beales (1978, Tables 1, B-3, B-6 and B-9), for 1977. Staff analysis of copyrighted Nielsen Media Research/Nielsen Monitor–Plus data; four weeks projected annually for 2004.

Note: Data from 1977 were adjusted to include 10 percent promos and PSAs in all categories to be comparable to the 2004 data. [a]Network ads include cable network and broadcast network ads. [b]Non-network ads include syndicated ads and local spots.

As a second approach to assess children's food ad exposure on all national shows, Table 5.4 presents the percent of advertising expenditures for food, along with children's food ad exposures for various types of shows available in the Abel study for 1977. Abel estimated national food advertising expenditures on all shows at 24.4 percent of all expenditures, as shown at the bottom of the table.[52] As can be seen from this data, children's food ad exposure is always a considerably higher percentage of the total than the comparable food ad spending percentage on all types of shows. Presumably, this is because the advertising time on shows more popular with children is less expensive on average than time on other shows. For instance, on shows with a 20 percent child audience share, 39.1 percent of ad expenditures are for food, but 57.7 percent of children's ad exposures are for food. The third column presents the ratio of children's food ad exposure percentages and food ad expenditures percentages for each type of show. The smallest differences are for the high child share shows (30 percent and 50 percent or more children in the audience), where the food ad exposure percentages are approximately 11 percent higher than the food ad expenditure percentages.

If we assume, conservatively, that the ratio of child ad exposure to ad expenditures on all national shows is equal to the lowest ratio found for the more general audience shows in the Abel data, that is, 1.36, we estimate that children's food ad exposure on all national shows is approximately 33.2 percent.[53]

Table 5.4. Percent Food Ad Expenditure versus Percent Children's Food Ad Exposure By Type of Show, Abel Study 1977

Type of Show	Percent Food Ad Expenditures	Percent Food Ad Exposure (2–11)	Ratio of Food Ad Exposures (2–11) to Expenditures
By Child Share			
20% Child Share	39.1	57.7	1.48
30% Child Share	54.1	59.9	1.11
50% Child Share	55.4	61.9	1.12
By Child Size			
≥ 3.5 million	30.1	47.1	1.56
≥ 5.0 million	30.5	46.1	1.51
≥ 8.0 million	29.2	39.5	1.36
All Shows	24.4		

Source: Abel (1978, Tables I, II, IV, VI, IX, XI, XIII, XVI, XVII, XVIII, XIX, and XX).

Children ages 2–11

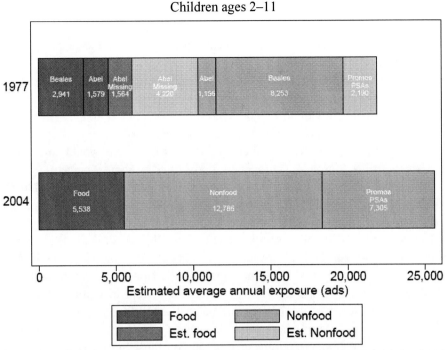

Source: Staff estimates based on Abel (1978, Tables XVI, XVII and XVIII), Beales (1978, Tables 1, B-3, B-6 and B-9), and Adler et al. (1977) for 1977. Staff analysis of copyrighted Nielsen Media Research/Nielsen Monitor–Plus data; four weeks projected annually for 2004.

Figure 5.1. Annual Exposure to TV Advertising: 1977 versus 2004.

These two approaches give us relatively similar measures of the potential magnitude of children's exposure to national food ads in 1977. To be conservative, we focus on the smaller of the two to draw out the implications for children's ad exposure; that is, we assume that approximately 33.2 percent of children's exposures from national ads were for food products, or 3,143 national food ads.[54] When added to the Beales estimate for local ads, this implies that children would have been exposed to 6,084 food ads overall in 1977.[55] Figure 5.1 illustrates.

The lower bar of Figure 5.1 shows children's estimated exposure to food ads, paid nonfood ads, and Promos and PSAs in 2004 — the horizontal width of the bar represents average annual exposure of 25,629 ads per year. The upper bar shows, from left to right, children's estimated food ad exposure from spot ads (Beales' data) and then their estimated food ad exposure from the subset of network shows analyzed by Abel. The third segment represents our estimate of children's exposure to food ads from the network shows excluded from Abel's analysis (1,564 food ads). The next segment represents the estimated exposure to nonfood ads from the excluded network shows (4,220 nonfood ads). The remaining segments show Abel's and Beales' estimates of children's exposure to nonfood ads and the Adler et al. (1977) estimate of exposure to Promos and PSAs. The overall horizontal width of the bar represents the Adler et al. (1977) estimate of the 1977 average annual exposure of 21,904 ads per year.

Thus, under this scenario, children's exposure to food ads would have fallen modestly since 1977, from 6,084 to 5,538 food ads, or by about 9 percent.[56]

While we believe this is a conservative and reasonable estimate of children's exposure to food ads in 1977, we also recognize that it is based on less detailed and specific data than the other estimates and analyses in this chapter. As a check on the core finding that children's exposure to food ads has not increased, we note from Table 5.4 that food ad spending on national network television is 24.4 percent of total ad spending on that medium in 1977. Note also from the table that for all the show groupings analyzed by Abel, the percent of children's food ad exposure is greater than the percent of food ad expenditure. We also see this pattern in the 2004 data, where food ad spending on network shows is 17.1 percent, while children's exposure to food ads on those shows is 22.6 percent. Together this evidence suggests, without any additional assumptions, that the proportion of children's national food ad exposure on all shows in 1977 should be greater than 24.4 percent, the percent of expenditure on food ads. Further, we can determine that children's national food ad exposure at any level above 27.4 percent of their total national ad exposure would imply a decrease in their exposure to food ads.[57] Therefore, it is only in the range where food ad exposure is between 24.4 percent and 27.4 percent that children's exposure to food ads could have plausibly increased since 1977. If food ad exposure were 27.4 percent of total ad exposure, the ratio of food ad exposure to food ad expenditure would have been 1.12, a ratio only seen on largely children's shows and greatly exceeded for all other show groupings.[58]

Thus, the available evidence indicates that children's exposure to food advertising has almost certainly declined since 1977, in our estimate by about 9 percent.

5.3. Changes in Exposure by Product Category

While coverage of the Abel data limits our ability to get precise estimates of children's ad exposure at the product category level in 1977, for most categories we can reasonably assess whether exposure has decreased or increased since 1977. For some categories, the exposure measured by Abel and Beales is greater than measured exposure for 2004 — clearly showing that if we had exposure for the "missing" shows, total exposure in 1977 must be greater than in 2004. For other categories, the exposure measured in 1977 is so much lower than that measured in 2004 that it is very likely that exposure was higher in 2004 than in 1977 — that is, the number of ads in that product category would have to be implausibly high in the "missing" shows for this not to be the case.

Table 5.5 gives children's ad exposure by product category from the various studies. The data indicates that children's exposure to TV ads for Cereal and Desserts and Sweets was lower in 2004 than in 1977. Children's 1977 exposure to Cereal ads on the programming analyzed by Abel and Beales was 1,064, while their exposure (on all shows) was 993 in 2004. Thus, even though we do not know the total exposure in 1977, it clearly has declined. We can apply similar reasoning to determine that children's exposure to ads for Desserts and Sweets has also declined. Children's 1977 exposure to ads for Desserts and Sweets on measured programming was 919, while their exposure on all shows was 898 in 2004.

Exposure to ads for Restaurants and Fast Food almost certainly increased. The 1977 exposure to Restaurants and Fast Food ads on this subset of shows was 745, compared to 1,367 on all shows in 2004. For exposure to have not increased, there must have been 622 ads in this category in the missing data, or 9.7 percent of all ad exposure on those programs. This seems unlikely given the percentage contribution of Restaurants and Fast Food in the data analyzed by Abel and Beales. We can apply similar reasoning to conclude that exposure to ads for Snacks has likely increased since 1977. The 1977 exposure to ads for Snacks on this subset of shows was 73, while the 2004 exposure on all shows was 490. If it were true that exposure to ads for Snacks had not increased, exposure on the missing shows must have been at least 417, or 6.5 percent of total exposure on those shows. Given their shares in the measured subset, this is implausible.

Abel (1978) and Beales (1978) provide insufficient information to determine how children's exposure to advertising in other food categories changed between 1977 and 2004.

Table 5.5. Children's Exposure to Advertising Product Categories: 1977 and 2004

Category	1977 Abel 20%+ Share		1977 Missing Estimated[d]		1977 Beales All Dayparts		2004 FTC All Ads	
	Ads	%	Ads	%	Ads	%	Ads	%
Cereal	595	19.6			469	3.8	993	3.9
Desserts and Sweets	373	12.3			546	4.4	898	3.5
Restaurants and Fast Food	113	3.7			632	5.1	1,367	5.3
Snacks	35	1.2			38	0.3	490	1.9
Dairy Products							353	1.4
Sweetened Drinks	62	2.0			273	2.2	430	1.7
Prepared Entrees							222	0.9
Other Food	401	13.2			984	7.9	786	3.1
All Food Products[a]	**1,579**	**52.0**	**1,564**	**26.8**	**2,941**	**23.7**	**5,539**	**21.6**
Games, Toys and Hobbies	610	20.1			1,359	10.9	1,909	7.4
Screen/Audio Entertainment							2,010	7.8
Bicycles; Sports and Exercise[b]					30	0.2	24	0.1
Promos and PSAs[c]	304	10.0	643	10.0	1,244	10.0	7,305	28.5
Other Non-food	546	18.0			6,864	55.2	8,842	34.5
All Non-food Products	**1,460**	**48.0**	**4,863**	**73.2**	**9,497**	**76.3**	**20,090**	**78.4**
Total	3,039		6,427		12,438		25,629	

Source: Staff estimates based on Abel (1978, Tables XVI, XVII, and XVIII), Beales (1978, Tables 1, B-3, B-6, B-9), and Adler et al. (1977) for 1977. Staff analysis of copyrighted Nielsen Media Research/Nielsen Monitor–Plus data; four weeks projected annually for 2004.

Note: [a]As a percentage of all ads (including Promos and PSAs), All Food Products in 1977 accounted for 52 percent in Abel's programs, 33 percent in the missing programs, and 24 percent in Beales' dayparts. [b]Bicycles for 1977, Sports and Exercise for 2004. [c]Promos and PSAs for 1977 estimated by Adler. [d]Estimated assuming that national food advertising constitutes 33.2 percent of all national advertising, as described in text.

Overall, it appears that the food ads children viewed in 2004 are more evenly spread over these food categories than in 1977. In 1977, ads for Cereal and Desserts and Sweets dominated children's food ad exposure. While these categories are relatively large in 2004, they are not nearly as dominant as in 1977.

Children's exposure to TV ads for Games, Toys and Hobbies was lower in 2004 than in 1977. Their 1977 exposure on measured shows was 1,969 while their total exposure to these ads was 1,909 in 2004. Children's exposure to Screen/Audio Entertainment ads was probably greater in 2004 than 1977. The components of this category that were advertised in 1977 were included in Other Nonfood in 1977 so we do not have baseline exposure for the category. However, we know that the first national TV ad campaigns for movies aired in 1975 ("Breakout" and "Jaws") and that the primary mode of advertising for movies in the 1970s was still newspapers.[59] Aside from Records, the other components are products that sold in small numbers, if at all, in 1977.[60] Therefore, we conclude that the exposure to ads in the Screen/Audio Entertainment category is likely substantially higher in 2004 than in 1977.

The 1977 studies examined Bicycles and found that children were exposed to few ads in that category. We chose a larger product category that includes Bicycles Sports and Exercise and found slightly lower exposure. Advertising for bicycles and sports equipment was a trivial part of the advertising children saw in 1977 and in 2004.

Children's exposure to Promos and PSAs was considerably higher in 2004 than in 1977. We cannot say how exposure to the PSA component changed between 1977 and 2004, because we do not have information on them separately in 1977. However, PSAs are a tiny portion of Promos and PSAs in 2004; they contribute less than 1 percent to Promos and PSAs' 28.5 percent. Thus, we can conclude that children's exposure to advertising for television programming (Promos) has increased substantially since 1977. Children's exposure to Other Nonfood ads was almost certainly greater in 2004 than in 1977. Their exposure to these ads on measured programming was 7,410 in 1977 and their exposure was 10,852 in 2004. (The 2004 number here includes the 1,922 Screen/Audio Entertainment exposures for comparability with the 1977 definition of Other Nonfood.)

5.4. Sources of Children's Ad Exposure in 1977 and 2004

A greater proportion of children's ad exposure is on children's shows in 2004. A direct comparison of our data from 2004 and the Abel and Beales analyses from 1977 makes it clear that children are getting a greater percentage of their ad exposure from children's programming in 2004. Table 5.6 summarizes our best estimates of children's ad exposures for food and nonfood products in the two years. Recall that the Beales analysis is for dayparts, rather than shows, so we cannot directly add the two 1977 analyses. Nonetheless, both parts of the 1977 analysis indicate that children were getting approximately one-quarter of their food ads from 50 percent child share shows or dayparts in 1977; in 2004, 50 percent of their food ad exposures came from 50 percent share shows.

In 1977 children got a substantial amount of their food advertising exposure on shows with between a 20 and 50 percent child audience share. As can be seen in Table 5.6 by comparing the fourth and sixth columns, adding family shows to children's shows more than doubles children's exposure to food advertising from non-network sources (60 percent versus 25 percent) and almost doubles it from network sources (50 versus 32 percent). In 2004 this is not the case; children's food ad exposure increases only modestly (from 50.4 percent to 63.5 percent) when we add family shows to children's shows.

Children's exposure to nonfood ads in 2004 is not as concentrated on children's programming as food ads, but the level is again higher than in 1977. About one-quarter of children's nonfood ad exposure is from children's shows in 2004, compared to 13 and 24 percent in the network and non-network analyses, respectively, in 1977.

Most children's ad exposure from children's programming was from cable shows in 2004; in 1977 most of their ad exposure was from broadcast network affiliates. Table 5.7 breaks out children's ad exposure for food and nonfood products in 2004 on broadcast and cable network shows, and on local spot and syndicated shows. As can be seen from the table, in 2004 most children's ad exposure from children's shows is from cable network programming; 2,726 of the 2,792 food ads, and 5,601 of the 5,881 nonfood ads seen on children's shows are from cable. Thus, in 2004, 97.6 percent of the food ads on children's shows are from cable programming as are 95.2 percent of nonfood ads.[61]

In 1977, over 90 percent of TV viewing was of broadcast network affiliates. Further, the ads on these affiliates was fairly balanced between national and local ads. As seen in Table 5.6, children were exposed to 993 food ads from network advertising on children's shows; they saw 735 food ads on children's dayparts from non-network ads. While not directly comparable, because of the show/daypart difference in the Abel and Beales' methodologies, it is clear that we do not see the heavy concentration in programming sources seen in the 2004 data. Nonfood advertising on 50 percent share dayparts is more concentrated in local ads, but again not to the level seen in 2004.

Thus, the evidence indicates a greater portion of children's ad exposure is on children's programs in 2004, and most of that is on cable networks.

Table 5.6. Ad Exposure From Children's Programming: 1977 versus 2004

	General[a]		Family[b]		Children[b]		Total
	Share 0-20%		Share 20-50%		Share ≥ 50%		
	Ads	%	Ads	%	Ads	%	Ads
1977							
Food							
Network (Abel)	1, 564	49.8	586	18.6	993	31.6	3, 143
Non-network (Beales)	1, 167	39.7	1, 039	35.3	735	25.0	2, 941
Nonfood[c]							
Network (Abel)	4, 863	76.9	671	10.6	789	12.5	6, 323
Non-network (Beales)	3,605	38.0	3,571	37.6	2,321	24.4	9,497
Total[c]							
Network (Abel)	6,427	67.9	1,257	13.3	1,782	18.8	9,466
Non-network (Beales)	4, 772	38.4	4, 610	37.1	3, 056	24.6	12,438
2004							
Food	2,023	36.5	723	13.1	2,792	50.4	5,538
Nonfood	11,568	57.6	2,942	14.6	5,581	27.8	20,091
Total	13,591	53.0	3,665	14.3	8,373	32.7	25,629

Source: Staff estimates based on Abel (1978, Tables XVI, XVII and XVIII), Beales (1978, Tables 1, B-3, B-6 and B-9), and Adler et al. (1977) for 1977. Staff analysis of copyrighted Nielsen Media Research/Nielsen Monitor–Plus data; four weeks projected annually for 2004.

Note: [a]Abel's "All Shows" figures are estimated as described in the previous section for shows missing in the Abel analysis. Network (Abel) is the sum of the first and third numerical columns in Table 5.5. [b]Ads from shows with between 20 percent and 50 percent of the audience made up of children 2–11 in the Abel 1977 network analysis and in the 2004 data, and from dayparts with between a 20 percent and 50 percent share in Beales 1977 non-network analysis. Ads from shows with at least 50 percent show or daypart share are defined similarly. [c]Nonfood and Total for 1977 include Promos and PSAs estimated at ten percent of total based on Adler et al. (1977).

6. CONCLUDING REMARKS

This study finds that children's exposure to television advertising has increased somewhat since 1977; however, their exposure to television food advertising has not increased over the same period and is likely to have fallen modestly. We also find that, due to changes in the television landscape, children are getting a substantial portion of their ad exposure from children's shows. In particular, children see about half of their TV food ads on children's programming. In this section we first summarize these and other key findings of our empirical analysis of children's exposure to television advertising. We then discuss how these findings relate to the potential role of television marketing in the prevalence of obesity in U.S. children. Finally, we draw out a few implications of this evidence for evaluating and guiding research on marketing to children.

Table 5.7. Children's Ad Exposure Sources in 2004

	All Shows		Share ≥ 20%		Share ≥ 50%	
	Ads	%	Ads	%	Ads	%
Food						
Cable Networks	985	15.5	3, 115	25.9	2, 726	31.4
Broadcast Networks	835	3.3	185	1.5	5	0.1
Syndicated	147	0.6	9	0.1	0	0.0
Local Spots	571	2.2	206	1.7	61	0.7
Total Food	5, 538	21.6	3, 515	29.2	2, 792	32.2
Nonfood						
Cable Networks	11,755	45.9	6,986	58.0	5,601	64.6
Broadcast Networks	792	18.7	651	5.4	40	0.5
Syndicated	606	2.4	17	0.1	0	0.0
Local Spots	2, 938	11.5	869	7.2	240	2.8
Total Nonfood	20, 091	78.4	8, 523	70.8	881	67.8
Total	25,629		12,038		8,673	

Source: Staff analysis of copyrighted Nielsen Media Research/Nielsen Monitor–Plus data; four weeks projected annually.

Note: Cable Networks and Broadcast Networks refer to exposure to advertising that originates with the national cable and broadcast networks, respectively. Syndicated refers to exposure to advertising that originates through national syndication while Local Spots refers to advertising that originates with the local affiliate.

6.1. Summary of Major Findings

6.1.1. Exposure to Television Advertising

In 2004 we estimate that children ages 211 saw about 25,600 television advertisements, 17 percent more than in 1977. Children saw about 18,300 paid advertisements in 2004, 7 percent less than in 1977; paid ads exclude promotional ads for television programming (and PSAs), and promotional ads grew substantially over this period. Children saw approximately 2 percent fewer minutes of advertising and 19 percent fewer minutes of paid advertising in 2004 than in 1977. Together, this evidence indicates that in 2004 children saw a larger number of ads overall, but fewer paid ads and fewer minutes of advertising than in 1977. These reductions reflect the combined impact of the reduced amount of time children spent watching ad-supported television in 2004 compared to 1977 and ads that are shorter on average than in 1977.

6.1.2. Exposure to Food Ads

Our study also developed estimates of children's exposure to food advertising. Children saw approximately 5,500 food ads in 2004, 22 percent of all ads viewed. The 1977 studies do not give us a complete estimate of children's exposure to food ads, but with reasonable assumptions from other data from the period, we conclude that children's food advertising exposure has not increased, and is likely to have fallen modestly.

In 1977 ads for Cereals and for Desserts and Sweets dominated children's food ad exposure, with the Restaurant and Fast Food and the Sweetened Drinks categories also among the top categories. In 2004 these categories are still among the top categories of food ads children see, though the Cereals and the Desserts and Sweets categories no longer dominate. Restaurant and Fast Food ads are probably at a higher level, and they are joined by Snacks and Dairy as substantial sources of children's food ad exposure. Thus, the mix of food advertisements seen by children in 2004 is somewhat more evenly spread across these food categories than in 1977.

6.1.3. Ads for Sedentary Pursuits

The reduction in food advertisements seen by children has been more than compensated for by increased Promotions for television programming and increased advertising for Screen and Audio Entertainment. These two categories have become major categories of advertising seen by children. Screen and Audio Entertainment now rivals Games, Toys and Hobbies as one of the leading nonfood categories of paid ads seen by children, and Promotions is three times as large as either. Together these facts imply that children saw nearly twice as many ads for sedentary pursuits as for food products in 2004.

6.1.4. Exposure to Ads on Children's Programming

A greater proportion of children's ad exposure is from children's programming in 2004. Children got approximately half of their food ad exposure from programs in which children are at least 50 percent of the audience in 2004, compared to about one quarter in 1977. Ads for some food categories appear to be targeted to children.[62] The relative importance of food ads on children's programming varies by food category. For instance, in 2004 children saw 80 percent of their Cereal ads on children's shows, but children saw only one-third of their Restaurant and Fast food ads there. In 2004 virtually all of the ad exposure from children's programming is from cable shows; in 1977, when cable programming was in its infancy, children's shows came from national broadcast and local sources.

6.1.5. When Children See Ads

Finally, our study presents evidence on when children get their television advertising exposure. Saturday morning is a popular viewing time for children, but children get almost as much advertising exposure from one weekday's primetime viewing (4.2 percent of the total) or from their Sunday primetime viewing (4.1 percent) as from Saturday morning (4.3 percent). Weekday viewing between 4 p.m. and 8 p.m. produces nearly as much advertising exposure per day as primetime (3.8 percent). Thus, children's television advertising exposure is not highly concentrated by time of day or day of the week. The viewing pattern for younger children (ages 2–5) differs from that for older children (ages 6–11) in that younger children get more of their exposure during daytime hours.

6.2. Discussion of Empirical Findings and Obesity

6.2.1. Evidence on TV Advertising's Relation to Obesity

Many commentators have suggested that marketing to children may be a significant factor in the growth of obesity in U.S. children.[63] This hypothesis is well beyond anything we could test formally with the data analyzed here, which is limited to television advertising. Nonetheless, our data can shed light on aspects of this hypothesized link.

First, our data do not support the view that children are exposed to more television food advertising today. Our primary scenario indicates that children's exposure to food advertising on television fell by about 9 percent between the 1977 studies and 2004. Children's exposure to all paid television advertising has fallen as well.

Second, our data do not support the view that children are seeing more advertising for low nutrition foods. In both years the food ads that children see are concentrated in the snacking, breakfast, and restaurant product areas. While the foods advertised on children's programming in 2004 do not constitute a balanced diet, this was the case as well in 1977, before the rise in obesity.

6.2.2. Evidence Related to Ad Restrictions on Children's Programming

Some have called for various restrictions on advertising to children, including a complete ban on advertising to younger children and further restrictions on the number of minutes of advertising on children's television programming. Others have called for self-regulation or legislation that would limit advertising on children's programming to foods that meet specified nutrition characteristics (CSPI 2005; IOM 2005; FTC/DHHS 2006). Some industry members have proposed voluntary commitments along these lines (CARU 2006). This chapter does not provide a basis to assess the likely effects of any of these approaches, or the substantial legal issues that would have to be addressed for regulation, but it does have several findings that relate to this discussion.

First, children today do get 50 percent of their food advertising from shows where children are at least 50 percent of the audience.[64] Thus, changes to the mix of ads on children's shows could have a nontrivial effect on the mix and number of food advertisements that children see. This effect would be considerably larger than would have been the case in 1977, when programming was not as specialized and children did not get much of their advertising exposure from children's programs. That said, children also get half of their food advertising exposure from nonchildren's shows and food advertising on those shows might increase if restrictions were placed on children's programming.

Second, our study does provide some insight on another issue that has received little attention in the public discussion: what type of advertising would likely replace restricted food advertising, if it is replaced? The hope is that advertising for better food might increase. Beyond that, the best guidance on this question is found by looking at the other products currently advertised on children's programs, since these are the products most likely to increase their advertising if food advertising is reduced. Currently, advertisements for sedentary entertainment products outnumber food advertisements by nearly two to one and constitute most of the other advertising on children's programming. Presumably these products would expand their advertising further, if food advertising were reduced. Whether such a shift in advertising seen by children would affect obesity in U.S. children either positively or negatively — is an open question that has received little attention.

Finally, it is worth noting that a restriction on advertising on children's programming would not fall evenly on industry participants. In 2004 broadcast networks had very few programs where children were more than 50 percent of the audience. Successful children's programming is now largely on children's cable networks. In fact, over 97 percent of food advertisements children see on children's shows are from cable programming.

Our study is limited to advertising on television. Television is still the medium where food advertisers spend most of their advertising dollars. In 2004 approximately 75 percent of all food advertising spending on measured media was spent on television, down from 83 percent in 1977 (BAR/LNA 1977, 2004). Many producers are exploring other advertising media and methods as television audiences become more expensive to reach. This is true for advertising to children as well. Advergaming, child-oriented producer-sponsored websites, product placements and other tie-ins with movies and television programming are all part of the marketing landscape, and research to quantify these efforts is only beginning (Moore 2006; FTC/DHHS 2006).[65]

6.3. Implications for Research on Marketing to Children

One of the key differences between this study and much of the literature is that the measured variable is exposure to advertising, a measure which takes account of how many children are in the audience for each ad aired on each show, based on very detailed Nielsen data. This exposure measure gives better estimates of how many and what type of ads children see on average, though obviously exposure is not the same as paying close attention to the ad. This exposure measure differs from other measures often used, such as the number of ads aired, which do not reflect the size of the audience seeing the ad.

A number of studies in the literature attempt to estimate the exposure measure from aggregate estimates, typically using measures of the number of ads on television per hour and the hours spent watching television (e.g. Adler et al. 1977; Chou et al. 2005; Kunkel and Gantz 1992; Gantz et al. 2007). As demonstrated in Section 3.1, footnote 19, these estimates can be quite close to the detailed exposure estimate if the component estimates are good; they can be very poor estimates if the component estimates are not appropriate for the audience of interest.

Some of the variation in estimates in the literature arises from the quality of these component estimates. For instance, we know that the amount of time children spend watching television is not the same as the amount of time spent watching ad-supported television. Public broadcasting and premium cable shows are not ad-supported television.[66] In 2004, approximately 70 percent of children's viewing was on ad-supported TV. If the total amount of television viewing time is used to estimate ad exposure, instead of the amount of ad- supported television, the estimate of exposure will be biased upward.

Also, the amount and type of advertising per hour varies by time of day, day of the week, and type of show. Estimates of the amount and type of advertising per hour can vary accordingly, depending on the sample of shows used to generate the estimate. The sample of shows must reasonably correspond to the viewing patterns of the audience of interest — children in our case — and must be appropriately weighted by viewing pattern for it to provide a good estimate of the number and type of ads seen by the audience. In many studies, researchers estimate ads seen by children by monitoring television on Saturday morning and sometimes during after-school hours. But as seen from this data, children get much of their advertising exposure from prime time television (more than 6 times as much as on Saturday mornings), and a sample that ignores this prime time programming will present a skewed view of children's ad exposure. Detailed data on time of viewing by children is presented in Appendix D to help guide future researchers.

6.4. Final Notes

This study was conducted to provide a comprehensive assessment of the amount and type of television advertising seen by children in 2004. It has been nearly 30 years since the last detailed evaluation of children's television ad exposure. Advertising seen by children has received considerable attention in recent years as a possible contributor to rising obesity in American children, and as a possible vehicle to help reverse that trend. Hopefully, this chapter will provide useful information to guide discussion of the issues. The chapter also provides a baseline against which to measure future changes in children's exposure to television advertising.

A. DATA AND METHODS

A.1. The Data

We investigate exposure to television advertising using a comprehensive database of advertising aired during four weeks in the 20032004 programming season. This data consists of copyrighted Nielsen Monitor-Plus/Nielsen Media

Research data linking Nielsen audience estimates to aired television advertising on monitored media. It covers all advertising aired on ad-supported television during the weeks of Nov. 2–8, 2003, Feb. 8–14, 2004, May 2–8, 2004, and July 4–10, 2004.[67] These weeks were chosen to match the Abel (1978) and Beales (1978) studies of children's exposure to television advertising and because they are in sweeps periods, the only time detailed local data is available.

The data include all television advertisements aired during the monitored programs, including paid advertisements, public service announcements (PSAs), and Promotions for a network's own or affiliated shows. The information provided for each ad include: the advertiser, the brand, the network, the program, the time the ad was aired, the length of the ad, the product category code, and estimates of viewership by those aged 6–11, 2–11, 12–17, and 18 and over.

We analyzed both national and local data. The national data covers advertising distributed by a national network or national syndicator and includes nearly one million ads. The local data covers spot advertising aired by broadcast network affiliates and independent stations in the 75 largest metropolitan markets and includes nearly five million spot ads. Spot ads are aired on a single affiliate or independent station (or several local stations in some cases).[68]

A.2. Assigning Ads to Product Categories

We use the product classification code (PCC) and brand category information for each ad to assign the ad to one of the 41 detailed product categories (see Table 3.4). The PCC identifies a particular family of products and the brand category further specifies the product within the class. For example, PCC F122 identifies cereal products. Within cereal products, the brand category distinguishes cereal (where the brand category is "cereal") from oatmeal (where the brand category is "oatmeal"). We rely on the PCC for initial classification and use the brand category when a PCC includes products belonging to more than one study category. For example, all advertisements for products with PCC G422 (noncomputerized games) are assigned to the Games, Toys, and Hobbies category; the brand category is not needed. However, PCC F144 contains advertisements for both bean products and rice products. In this case, we assign products where the brand category is "beans" or "tofu" to Vegetables and Legumes and products where the brand category is "couscous" or "rice" to the Other Food category.

In most cases, the combination of PCC and brand category are sufficient to assign a product to one of the study categories. However, the PCC and brand category cannot distinguish between regular and highly-sugared cereals, for example. In cases such as these, we also use nutritional data collected from product labels and the USDA National Nutrient Database.[69] The use of nutritional information in assigning ads to product categories is described in the "Other Criteria" column of Table B.1. For example, the PCC and brand categories containing pure fruit juices also contain fruit drinks; an ad was assigned to Fruit Juices only if nutritional information for the product indicated it was 100 percent juice.[70]

A.3. Estimating Exposure to Television Advertising

The audience estimates in the data are expressed as Gross Ratings Points (GRPs) — the percentage of a given population (U.S. population or population of a given metropolitan area) watching a program or advertisement. Multiplying the audience estimate in GRPs for a given ad by the appropriate population figure yields the estimated number of viewers exposed to the ad. We calculate total population exposure by summing the estimated number of viewers over all advertising. Average exposure is obtained by dividing by the population figure.[71] This process is carried out separately on the national data and each of the 75 metropolitan areas. Then we use a weighted average of the local average exposure figures as a nationally representative measure of average exposure to spot ads. This weighted average exposure is added to national exposure to obtain our final average exposure estimate. To project annually, we multiply the estimated exposure by 365/28.

We estimate exposure to television advertising for a given product category by carrying out a similar procedure, restricted to ads in that product category.

A.4. Estimating Daily Television Viewing Habits

We also use GRPs to calculate the average amount time children spend watching ad- supported TV each day. We divide each day into 30 minute blocks of time and calculate the average audience in each block for each network, as described above. We use 30 minute blocks of time since many programs air for a multiple of 30 minutes. We multiply the average audience for each 30 minute block by 30 minutes to estimate the total number of person-minutes in each block. We then aggregate over the day to get the total number of person-minutes viewed per day and divide by the appropriate population estimate to compute the average number of minutes viewed by a person in that age group. We combine national and local data as in the procedure used to calculate exposure to advertising.

B. Definition of Categories

Table B.1 details the product classification codes (PCCs) and Nielsen brand categories assigned to each FTC product category. The table omits the PCCs and brand categories assigned to Other Nonfood; any PCC or brand category not otherwise assigned is assigned to Other Nonfood.[72] The most prevalent advertisements assigned to Other NonFood include those for department stores, automobiles, telecommunications services, and financial services. Other prominent examples include household cleaning supplies, travel services, and toiletries.

When we require information in addition to the PCC and brand category to distinguish between one or more FTC study categories, the extra criteria are listed in parenthesis in the "Other criteria" column. Brand categories in *italics* indicate those categories actually present in the data; brand categories not so emphasized come from Nielsen's master list, but do not appear in our data. PCCs marked with a '*' represent PCCs in which brand categories are split between one or more FTC product categories. Sometimes the brand category in the data does not exactly match the brand category in the Nielsen master list (e.g. PCC code F212 contains a product category 'SNACK BAR' in the data, but 'SNACK BARS' in the Nielsen master list). In these situations, the table lists the brand category present in the data followed by the brand category from the master list in brackets.

C. What is Advertised to Children: Detailed Findings C.1 Children, 2–11

Table C.1 presents findings related to those presented in Section 3.3. It shows how exposure to advertising at the detailed category level changes as the share of children changes.

Table B.1. FTC product categories

FTC Category	Nielsen PCC	Nielsen brand category	Other criteria
Regular Cereal	F122*	CEREAL, FIBER TOPPING, OATMEAL, WEBSITE-CEREAL	(≤ 30% sugar by weight)
Highly Sugared Cereal	F122*	CEREAL, OATMEAL	(> 30% sugar by weight)
Beer, Wine and Mixers	F316	BEER, BEER PDTS, BEER-NON ALCOHOLIC, WEBSITE-BEER, WEBSITE-BEER PDTS	
	F330	CHAMPAGNE, WINE, WINE COOLER	
	F330	BEVERAGES-ALCOHOLIC, BOURBON WHISKEY, BRANDY-COGNAC, CANADIAN WHISKEY, GIN, IRISH WHISKEY, LIQUEUR, LIQUOR, RUM, SCOTCH WHISKEY, TEQUILA, VODKA, WEBSITE-LIQUOR, WEBSITE-RETAIL LIQUOR, WEBSITE-WINE, WHISKEY	
	F340	COCKTAIL MIXES	
Desserts and Dessert Ingredients	F113*	BAKING CHOCOLATE, BAKING MIX, BROWNIE MIX, BUTTERSCOTCH MORSELS, CAKE DECORATIONS, CAKE MIX, CANDY APPLE KIT, CHEESECAKE MIX, CHOCOLATE MORSELS, COOKIE DOUGH, COOKIE MIX, FOOD COLORING, FROSTING, MINT MORSELS, MORSELS, PEANUT BUTTER MORSELS, PIE CRUST, PIE FILLLING, PIE MIX, SHREDDED COCONUT, VANILLA MORSELS	
	F115	GELATIN-MIX, GELATIN-PREPARED, MOUSSE DESSERT, PUDDING-MIX, PUDDING-PREPARED	
	F129	FRUIT TOPPINGS, ICE CREAM TOPPINGS, WHIPPED TOPPING	
Candy	F211*	CANDY, CANDY BAR, CANDY PDTS, MARSHMALOWS, WEBSITE-CANDY	
	G719*	STORE-CANDY	
Appetizers, Snacks and Nuts	F212*	CORN CHIPS, NUTS, POPCORN, POPPING CORN, POTATO CHIPS, PRETZELS, SNACKS, TORTILLA CHIPS, WEBSITE-NUTS, WEBSITE-SNACKS	
Regular Non-carbonated Beverages	F171*	ICED COFFEE, ICED TEA	(Non-carbonated drink not advertised as diet or reduced calorie nor 100% juice.)
	F172*	DRINK MIX, DRINK MIX-ISOTONIC, DRINK PDTS, DRINKS-ISOTONIC, FRUIT DRINK PDTS, FRUIT DRINKS, FRUIT JUICES, WEBSITE-DRINK PDTS, WEBSITE-FRUIT JUICES	
	F173*	VEGETABLE JUICE	

Table B.1. Continued

FTC Category	Nielsen PCC	Nielsen brand category	Other criteria
	F223*	DRINKS-NON CARBONATED, MILK SHAKE	
Diet Non-carbonated Beverages	F172*	FRUIT JUICES	(Advertised as diet or reduced calorie, generally artificially sweetened)
	F223*	DRINKS-NON CARBONATED	
Fruit Juices	F172*	FRUIT DRINKS, FRUIT JUICES	(100% juice)
	F173*	VEGETABLE JUICE	
Cakes, Pies and Pastries	F162	BROWNIES, CAKES, CHEESECAKE, CUPCAKES, DESSERTS, DOUGHNUTS, PASTRY, PIES, SNACK CAKES	
Crackers	F163*	CRACKERS, POPCORN CAKES, RICE CAKES	
Snack, Granola and Cereal Bars	F212*	SNACK BAR [SNACK BARS]	
Regular Gum	F211*	CHEWING GUM, WEBSITE-CHEWING GUM	(All other gums.)
Sugarless Gum	F211*	CHEWING GUM	(Sugarless according to product label.)
Cookies	F163*	COOKIES	
Regular Carbonated Beverages	F221	CLUB SODA, REG SOFT DRINK, SELITZER WATER, SOFT DRINKS, TONIC WATER, WEBSITE-SOFT DRINKS	
Diet Carbonated Beverages	F222	DIET SOFT DRINK	
Restaurants and Fast Food	G330*	RESTAURANT, RESTAURANT-QUICK SVC, WEBSITE-REST-QUICK SVC [WEBSITE-RESTAURANT-QUICK SVC], WEBSITE-RESTAURANT	
Raisins and Other Dried Fruit	F142*	RAISINS	
Ice Cream	F133	CONES-ICE CREAM, FROZEN DESSERT, FROZEN DESSERT PDTS, FROZEN JUICE NOVELTIES, FROZEN NOVELTIES, FROZEN YOGURT, ICE, ICE CREAM, ICE CREAM NOVELTIES, ICE MILK, SHERBET, SORBET, WEBSITE-FROZEN NOVELTIES	
	G716*	STORE-ICE CREAM	
Fresh Fruit	F141	FRUIT-CITRUS	

FTC Category	Nielsen PCC	Nielsen brand category	Other criteria
	F 142*	FRUIT-NON CITRUS	
Prepared Entrees	F 125*	PASTA DINNERS	
	F 126*	CHILI, ENTREES-FROZEN, ENTREES-PREPARED, HASH, ORIENTAL NOODLES, RICE MIX, WEBSITE-ENTREES-FROZEN	
Frozen Pizza	F 126*	PIZZA-FROZEN, PIZZA-REFRIG	
Dairy Products and Substitutes	F 131	BUTTER, BUTTERMILK, CREAM, EGGNOG, EGGS, MILK, PROCESSED EGG	
	F 132	CHEESE, CREAM CHEESE	
	F 134	NON-DAIRY CREAMER	
	F 139	COTTAGE CHEESE, DAIRY PDTS, SOUR CREAM, YOGURT	
Vegetables and Legumes	F 143	FRENCH FRIES, HASH BROWNS, OLIVES, PRODUCE, SALADS, SAUERKRAUT, VEGETABLES, VEGETABLES-CANNED, VEGETABLES-FRESH, VEGETABLES-FROZEN	
	F 144*	BEANS, TOFU	
Meat, Poultry and Fish	F 150	BACON, BEEF, HOT DOGS [HOT DOG], LAMB, LUNCHEON MEAT, MEAT, MEAT PDTS, PORK, POULTRY, SAUSAGE, SEAFOOD, WEBSITE-SEAFOOD	
Bread, Rolls, Waffles and Pan-cakes	F 161	BAGELS, BREAD, BREADSTICKS, BUNS, CROSSANTS, DOUGH, ENGLISH MUFFINS, FRENCH TOAST-FROZEN, MUFFINS, PANCAKES-FROZEN, ROLLS, TACO SHELLS, TORTILLAS, WAFFLES-FROZEN	
Other Food and Beverage	F 111	ARTIFICIAL SWEETENER, HONEY, SUGAR, SYRUP	
	F 112	BUTTER-MARGARINE BLEND, COOKING OIL, LARD, MARGARINE, NON-STICK SPRAY, SHORTENING	
	F 113*	BREAD MIX, CORNMEAL, FLOUR, MUFFIN MIX, PANCAKE-WAFFLE MIX, PIZZA CRUST, WEBSITE-YEAST, YEAST	
	F 114	CLAM JUICE, COOKING WINE, FLAVORING, MARINADE, SALT, SEASONING, SEASONING MIX, VINEGAR	

Table B.1. Continued

FTC Category	Nielsen PCC	Nielsen brand category	Other criteria
	F116	APPLE SAUCE, HORSERADISH, KETCHUP, MUSTARD, PICKLES, RELISH	
	F117	CRANBERRY SAUCE, DIPS, GRAVY, GRAVY MIX, PASTA SAUCE, SALSA, SAUCE, SAUCE-BARBECUE, SAUCE-COCKTAIL, SAUCE-HOT, SAUCE-MIX, SAUCE-ORIENTAL, SAUCE-PICANTE, SAUCE-POULTRY, SAUCE-SOY, SAUCE-STEAK, SAUCE-STIR-FRY, SAUCE-TARTAR, SAUCE-TERIYAKI, SAUCE-WORCESTERSHIRE, TOMATO PASTE	
	F118	MAYONNAISE, SALAD DRESSINGS, SALAD DRESSINGS-BOTTLED, SALAD DRESSINGS-MIX	
	F119	BACON BITS, BAKING PWDR, BAKING SODA, BREAD CRUMBS, COATING MIX, CORN STARCH, CROUTONS, FAT SUBSTITUTE, FRUIT PECTIN, PRESERVATIVE, STUFFING MIX	
	F121	SOUP, SOUP-CONDENSED, SOUP-MIX, SOUP-RTS	
	F124	BABY FOODS [BABY FODS], INFANT FORMULA, WEBSITE-BABY FOODS	
	F125*	PASTA	
	F128	FRUIT SPREADS, JAMS & JELLIES, PEANUT BUTTER, PRESERVES, SANDWICH SPREAD	
	F144*	COUSCOUS, RICE, WEBSITE-RICE	
	F171*	CHOCOLATE SYRUP, COCOA, COCOA MIX, COFFEE, COFFEE-BEAN-CAF, COFFEE-GROUND-CAF, COFFEE-GROUND-DECAF, COFFEE-INSTANT-CAF, COFFEE-INSTANT-DECAF, HOT COCOA MIX, ICED TEA MIX, TEAS, WEBSITE-COFFEE	
	F190	FOOD PDTS, WEBSITE-FOOD PDTS	
	F211*	BREATH MINTS, CHEWING GUM, WEBSITE-BREATH MINTS	
	F224	BOTTLED WATER, MINERAL WATER, WEBSITE-BOTTLED WATER	
	G716*	BAKERY, FOOD DISTRIBUTOR, SHOP-BAGEL, SHOP-DOUGHNUT, STORE-BEVERAGES, STORE-COFFEE-TEA, STORE-FOOD, STORE-FROZEN YOGURT, STORE-HEALTH FOOD, STORE-LIQUOR, STORE-MEAT-SEAFOOD, STORE-POPCORN, STORE-PRODUCE, SUPERMAR-KET, WEBSITE-BAKERY, WEBSITE-HEALTH FOODS, WEBSITE-RETAIL BEVERAGES, WEBSITE-RETAIL COFFEE-TEA, WEBSITE-RETAIL FOOD, WEBSITE-RETAIL HLTH FOOD, WEBSITE-RETAIL MEAT-SEAFD, WEBSITE-RETAIL PRODUCE, WEBSITE-SUPERMARKET	

FTC Category	Nielsen PCC	Nielsen brand category	Other criteria
Games, Toys and Hobbies	G-422	CARDS-NOVELTY, GAME, GAME-BOARD, GAME-CARD, PLAYING CARDS, *POOL TABLES*, PUZZLE, *SWING SETS*, WEBSITE-CARDS-NOVELTY, WEBSITE-GAME-BOARD, *WEBSITE-GAMES*	
	G-423	BUILDING KITS, *BUILDING SETS*, COLORING BOOKS, CRAYONS, *PLAYSETS*, *RACE SET*, *RIDEABLE TOYS*, SKATEBOARDS, *STUFFED TOYS*, *TOY ACCESS*, *TOY FIGURES-DOLLS*, TOY INSTRUMENTS, *TOY VEHICLES*, TOY VEHICLES-RADIO CONTROL [TOY VEHICLES-RADIO CONTROL], *TOYS*, TRAIN SET, *WEBSITE-TOYS*	
	G-424	CALLIGRAPHY KIT, COLORING KIT, *CRAFT SUPLS*, DRAWING KIT, *MODEL KITS*, PAINT SET	
	G-717*	*STORE-ARTS & CRAFTS*, *STORE-HOBBY*, *STORE-PLAYGROUND SETS*, *STORE-TOYS*, WEBSITE-PLAYGROUND SETS, WEBSITE-RETAIL ART & CRFT, WEBSITE-RETAIL HOBBY, WEBSITE-RETAIL TOYS	
Screen / Audio Entertainment	G-310	*MOTION PICTURE*, WEBSITE-MOTION PICTURE	
	G-421	COMPUTER TOY, ENTERTAINMENT SFTWRE, GAME-VCR, GAME-VCR-DVD, *GAME-VIDEO ACCESS*, GAME-VIDEO SYS, VIDEO GAME-CLUB, WEBSITE-ENTRTNMNT SFTWRE, WEBSITE-GAME-VIDEO ACCESS, WEBSITE-GAME-VIDEO SYS	
	G-719*	*STORE-RECORDS-TAPES-CDS*, *STORE-VIDEO*, WEBSITE-RECORDS-TAPES-CDS, *WEBSITE-RETAIL ENT SFTWRE*, WEBSITE-RETAIL VIDEO	
	H-331	BOOKS-RECORDINGS, RECORDINGS, RECORDINGS-AUDIO, WEBSITE-RECORDINGS AUDIO	
	H-332	*RECORDINGS-VIDEO*, WEBSITE-RECORDINGS-VIDEO	
	R-100*	*RECORDINGS-AUDIO-DIR RESP*, *RECORDINGS-DIR RESP*, *RECORDINGS-VIDEO-DIR RESP*	
Dental Supplies	D-121	*BREATH FRESHENER*, DENTAL FLOSS, DENTAL PSTS, *DENTAL RINSE*, *DENTURE ADHESIVE*, DENTURE CLEANER, MOUTHWASH, TOOTH POLISH, TOOTH PWDR, *TOOTHBRUSH*, TOOTHBRUSH-ELECTRIC [PCC originally D150], *TOOTHPASTE-GEL*, WEBSITE-MOUTHWASH, WEBSITE-TOOTHPASTE-GEL	
Sporting Goods	B-119*	*BOAT RENTAL SVCS*	

Table B.1. Continued

FTC Category	Nielsen PCC	Nielsen brand category	Other criteria
	G411	FISH TRACKER, FISHING EQUIP, FISHING LINE, FISHING REEL, FISHING ROD, FISHING TACKLE, TACKLE BOX, WEBSITE-FISHING EQUIP	
	G412	AMMUNITION, FIREARM ACCESS, FIREARMS, FIREWORKS, RIFLES, SHOTGUNS	
	G413	BATTERIES-BOAT, BOAT DLRSHP, BOAT TRAILERS, BOATING EQUIP, BOATS, INBOARD MOTOR, INFLATABLE BOATS, MARINA, MARINE ENGINES, OUTBOARD MOTOR, SHOP-BOAT REPAIR, TROLLING MOTOR, WEBSITE-BOAT DLRSHP, WEBSITE-BOATING EQUIP, WEBSITE-BOATS	
	G415	BICYCLE ACCESS, BICYCLES	
	G416	SKIING EQUIP [SKIING EQUIPMENT], SKIS-SNOW, SKIS-WATER, SNOWBOARD	
	G417	GOLF BAGS, GOLF BALLS, GOLF CARTS, GOLF CLUBS, GOLF EQUIP, WEBSITE-GOLF EQUIP-MENT	
	G418	TENNIS BALLS, TENNIS EQUIP, TENNIS RACQUETS	
	G419	ARCHERY EQUIPMENT, BASEBALL EQUIP, BASEBALL GLOVE, BASEBALLS, BASKETBALL EQUIP, BASKETBALLS, BOWLING BALLS, BOWLING EQUIP, CAMPING EQUIP, CAMPING TENTS, FOOTBALL EQUIP, FOOTBALLS, HOCKEY EQUIP, HOCKEY STICKS, HUNTING BOWS, HUNTING EQUIP, ICE CHEST, ICE SKATES, IN-LINE SKATES, ROLLER SKATES, SLEEPING BAGS, SNORKEL-MASK, SPORTING EQUIP, SURFBOARD, SWIM FINS, TRAMPO-LINE, WATER SAFETY DEVICE, WEBSITE-SPORTING GOODS	
	G717*	STORE-SPORTING GOODS, WEBSITE-RETAIL SPRING GDS	
	G719*	STORE-BICYCLES, STORE-BILLIARDS	
Exercise Equipment	D242	EXERCISE EQUIP, WEBSITE-EXERCISE EQUIP, WEBSITE-RETAIL EXRCSE EQP	
	G719*	STORE-EXERCISE EQUIP	
	R109*	EXERCISE EQUIP-DIR RESP	
Diets and Diet Aids	D217	REDUCING AIDS, WEBSITE-REDUCING AIDS	

FTC Category	Nielsen PCC	Nielsen brand category	Other criteria
	D241	*FITNESS CTRS-CLUBS, FITNESS PROGRAMS, GYMNASTIC CTR, HEALTH CARE PROGRAM, WEBSITE-FITNESS CTRS-CLBS, WEBSITE-WEIGHT LOSS CTR, WEBSITE-WEIGHT LOSS PROGM, WEIGHT LOSS CTR, WEIGHT LOSS PROGRAM*	
Footwear	A131	*BOOTS, SHOES, SLIPPERS, WEBSITE-SHOES*	
	A132	*BOWLING SHOES, GOLF SHOES, PROTECTIVE FOOTWEAR, SKI BOOTS, SPORTING FOOTWEAR, WEBSITE-SPORTING FOOTWEAR*	
	G711*	*STORE-SHOES*	
Computer Hardware and Internet Service	B143*	*INTERNET SVC PROVIDER, INTERNET SVCS, WEBSITE-INTERNET SVC PRVD, WEBSITE-INTERNET SVCS*	
	B311*	*COMPUTER ACCESSORIES [COMPUTER ACCESSSORIES], COMPUTER HARDWARE, COMPUTER MONITORS, COMPUTER PERIPHERALS, COMPUTER SYS, COMPUTERS-HAND HELD, MODEMS, OFFICE AUTOMATION SYS, PRINTERS, WEBSITE-COMPUTER HARDWARE, WEBSITE-COMPUTER PERPHRLS, WEBSITE-COMPUTER SYS, WEBSITE-COMPUTERS, WORD PROCESSORS*	
	G715*	*STORE-COMPUTERS*	
Computer Software (Non-game)	B340	*COMPUTER SFTWRE, WEBSITE-COMPUTER SFTWRE*	
	G715*	*STORE-COMPUTER SFTWRE*	

Table B.1. Continued

FTC Category	Nielsen PCC	Nielsen brand category	Other criteria
Promos	PXXX	PROMO, TV PGM-MORNING-SPORTS, TV PGM-MORNING-TALK SHOW, TV PGM-MORNING-NEWS, TV PGM-MORNING-ENT, TV PGM-MULTI-ENT, TV PGM-DAYTIME-SPORTS, TV PGM-DAYTIME-TALK SHOW, TV PGM-DAYTIME-NEWS, TV PGM-DAYTIME-ENT, TV PGM-EVENING-SPORTS, TV PGM-EVENING-TALK SHOW, TV PGM-EVENING-NEWS, TV PGM-EVENING-ENT, TV PGM-PRIME-SPORTS, TV PGM-PRIME-TALK SHOW, TV PGM-PRIME-NEWS, TV PGM-PRIME-ENT, TV PGM-LATENITE-SPORTS, TV PGM-LATENITE-TALK SHOW, TV PGM-LATENITE-NEWS, TV PGM-LATENITE-ENT, TV PGM-OVERNITE-SPORTS, TV PGM-OVERNITE-TALK SHOW, TV PGM-OVERNITE-NEWS, TV PGM-OVERNITE-ENT; TV PGM-MULTI-SPORTS, TV PGM-MULTI-NEWS, TV PGM-MULTI-ENT, TV PGM-SYND-SPORTS, TV PGM-SYND-TALK SHOW, TV PGM-SYND-NEWS, TV PGM-SYND-ENT, TV PGM-CABLE-SPORTS, TV PGM-CABLE-TALK SHOW, TV PGM-CABLE-NEWS, TV PGM-CABLE-ENT, BROAD-CAST TV NETWORK, CABLE TV NETWORK, HISPANIC TV NETWORK, TV STATION	(classification based on Nielsen flag identifying promos)
PSAs	B182	PSA, WEBSITE-PSA	(classification based on Nielsen flag identifying promos)
	G900*	VIGNETTE	
Over-the-counter Medication	D211	ASPIRIN, PAIN RELIEVING RUB, PAIN RELVR, SLEEPING AID, WEBSITE-PAIN RELIEVERS	
	D212	ALLERGY REMEDY, ASTHMA MEDICATION, COLD REMEDIES, COLD REMEDIES-MULTI SYMP, COUGH REMEDIES, NASAL DECONGESTANTS, SINUS MEDICATIONS, THROAT REME-DIES	
	D213	ANTACIDS, DIARRHEA MEDICATION, DIGESTIVE AID, WEBSITE-ANTACIDS	
	D214	LAXATIVES	
	D215	CALCIUM SUPPLMT, NUTRITIONAL PDTS, NUTRITIONAL SUPPLMT, VITAMINS, WEBSITE-NUTRITIONAL SUPPLMT	
	D216	LIP MEDICATION, SKIN TREATMENTS-MED	
	D219	EAR MEDICATION, EYE DROPS, EYE MEDICATION, FOOT CARE-MED, HEMORRHOIDAL REMEDY, INSECT REPELLENT, MOTION SICKNESS REMEDY, ORAL REMEDY, SMOKING DETERRENT, STIMULANTS, WART REMEDY, WATER LOSS REMEDY, WATER RETENTION REMEDY, WEBSITE-FOOT CARE-MED, WEBSITE-SMOKING DETERRENT	

FTC Category	Nielsen PCC	Nielsen brand category	Other criteria
Prescription Medication	D218*	*PHARMACEUTICAL HOUSES*, *PRESCRIPTION DRUGS-HUMAN*, WEBSITE-PHRMCUTCL HOUSES, WEBSITE-PRSCRPTN DRG-HMN	
Other Nonfood Advertising	—	All product codes and product categories not categorized elsewhere	

Brand categories in italics are present in the data. PCC codes and brand categories in brackets list the corresponding entry from the master list when there is a discrepancy.

*At least one of the brand categories associated with the PCC is assigned to another study category.

Table C.1. Detailed Annual Exposure to TV Advertising by Audience Share

Children ages 2–11

Category	All ads		Share ≥ 20%		Share ≥ 50%	
	Ads	%	Ads	%	Ads	%
Regular Cereal	157	0.6	88	0.7	70	0.8
Highly Sugared Cereal	836	3.3	800	6.6	712	8.2
Candy	468	1.8	318	2.6	244	2.8
Desserts and Dessert Ingredients	52	0.2	30	0.3	25	0.3
Cakes, Pies and Pastries	94	0.4	89	0.7	76	0.9
Regular Gum	104	0.4	79	0.7	59	0.7
Cookies	166	0.6	131	1.1	112	1.3
Ice Cream	15	0.1	7	0.1	4	0.0
Restaurants and Fast Food	1,367	5.3	656	5.5	436	5.0
Appetizers, Snacks and Nuts	343	1.3	290	2.4	259	3.0
Crackers	99	0.4	79	0.7	68	0.8
Snack, Granola and Cereal Bars	48	0.2	20	0.2	13	0.2
Dairy Products and Substitutes	353	1.4	271	2.3	239	2.8
Regular Carbonated Beverages	147	0.6	43	0.4	18	0.2
Regular Non-carbonated Beverages	283	1.1	191	1.6	144	1.7
Prepared Entrees	205	0.8	138	1.1	112	1.3
Frozen Pizza	17	0.1	3	0.0	1	0.0
Beer, Wine and Mixers	132	0.5	5	0.0	0	0.0
Diet Carbonated Beverages	20	0.1	2	0.0	0	0.0
Diet Non-carbonated Beverages	17	0.1	3	0.0	0	0.0
Fruit Juices	51	0.2	7	0.1	0	0.0
Sugarless Gum	25	0.1	6	0.1	4	0.0
Canned Fruit	0	0.0	0	0.0	0	0.0
Raisins and Other Dried Fruit	0	0.0	0	0.0	0	0.0
Fresh Fruit	0	0.0	0	0.0	0	0.0
Vegetables and Legumes	16	0.1	3	0.0	0	0.0
Meat, Poultry and Fish	48	0.2	7	0.1	0	0.0
Bread, Rolls, Waffles and Pancakes	155	0.6	127	1.1	107	1.2
Other Food and Beverage	322	1.3	120	1.0	86	1.0
All Food Products	5,538	21.6	3,515	29.2	2,792	32.2
Games, Toys and Hobbies	1,909	7.5	1,827	15.2	1,629	18.8
Screen / Audio Entertainment	2,010	7.8	1,205	10.0	888	10.2
Sporting Goods	23	0.1	16	0.1	12	0.1
Exercise Equipment	1	0.0	0	0.0	0	0.0
Promos	7,097	27.7	3,432	28.5	2,395	27.6
PSAs	208	0.8	120	1.0	79	0.9

Table C.1. Continued

Category	All ads		Share ≥ 20%		Share ≥ 50%	
	Ads	%	Ads	%	Ads	%
Dental Supplies	220	0.9	55	0.5	38	0.4
Diets and Diet Aids	64	0.2	8	0.1	1	0.0
Footwear	111	0.4	54	0.4	36	0.4
Computer Hardware and Internet Services	230	0.9	75	0.6	49	0.6
Computer Software (Non-game)	13	0.0	0	0.0	0	0.0
Over-the-counter Medication	648	2.5	95	0.8	24	0.3
Prescription Medication	312	1.2	34	0.3	4	0.1
Other Nonfood Advertising	7,244	28.3	1,602	13.3	727	8.4
All Nonfood Products	20,091	78.4	8,523	70.8	5,881	67.8
Total	25,629		12,038		8,673	

Source: Staff analysis of copyrighted Nielsen Media Research/Nielsen Monitor–Plus data; four weeks projected annually.

Younger children ages 2–5

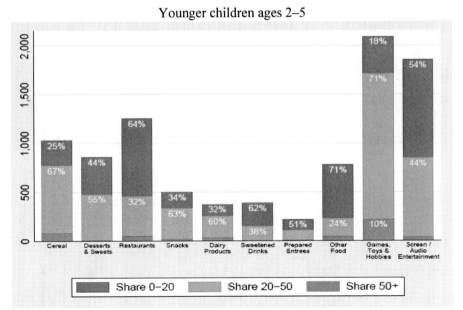

Source: Staff analysis of copyrighted Nielsen Media Research/Nielsen Monitor{Plus data; four weeks projected annually.

Note: Promos and PSAs and Other Nonfood Advertising omitted because they dominate the graph.

Figure C.1. Annual Exposure to TV Advertising, Selected Categories.

C.2. Younger Children, 2–5

This section provides additional findings related to those presented in Section 3.6. First, a graph shows exposure to selected categories of ads on general programming, family shows, and children's shows. Tables presenting findings at a more detailed category level follow.

Table C.2. Annual Exposure to TV Advertising By Product Category

Younger children ages 2–5

Category	Ads	%	Detailed category	Ads	%
Cereal	1,031	4.1	Regular Cereal	160	0.6
			Highly Sugared Cereal	871	3.5
Desserts and Sweets	857	3.4	Candy	441	1.8
			Desserts and Dessert Ingredients	51	0.2
			Cakes, Pies and Pastries	95	0.4
			Regular Gum	96	0.4
			Cookies	160	0.6
			Ice Cream	14	0.1
Restaurants and Fast Food	1,252	5.0	Restaurants and Fast Food	1,252	5.0
Snacks	499	2.0	Appetizers, Snacks and Nuts	354	1.4
			Crackers	101	0.4
			Snack, Granola and Cereal Bars	44	0.2
Dairy Products	370	1.5	Dairy Products and Substitutes	370	1.5
Sweetened Drinks	388	1.6	Regular Carbonated Beverages	127	0.5
			Regular Non-carbonated Beverages	261	1.0
Prepared Entrees	218	0.9	Prepared Entrees	203	0.8
			Frozen Pizza	15	0.1
Other Food	776	3.1	Beer, Wine and Mixers	116	0.5
			Diet Carbonated Beverages	19	0.1
			Diet Non-carbonated Beverages	15	0.1
			Fruit Juices	51	0.2

Table C.2. Continued

Category	Ads	%	Detailed category	Ads	%
			Sugarless Gum	23	0.1
			Canned Fruit	0	0.0
			Raisins and Other Dried Fruit	0	0.0
			Fresh Fruit	0	0.0
			Vegetables and Legumes	15	0.1
			Meat, Poultry and Fish	44	0.2
			Bread, Rolls, Waffles and Pancakes	155	0.6
			Other Food and Beverage	338	1.4
All Food Products	**5,390**	**21.6**	**All Food Products**	**5,390**	**21.6**
Games, Toys and Hobbies	2,092	8.4	Games, Toys and Hobbies	2,092	8.4
Screen / Audio Entertainment	1,853	7.4	Screen / Audio Entertainment	1,853	7.4
Sports and Exercise	21	0.1	Sporting Goods	21	0.1
			Exercise Equipment	0	0.0
Promos and PSAs	7,270	29.2	Promos	7,065	28.3
			PSAs	205	0.8
Other Nonfood	8,314	33.3	Dental Supplies	240	1.0
			Diets and Diet Aids	58	0.2
			Footwear	99	0.4
			Computer Hardware and Internet Services	215	0.9
			Computer Software (Non-game)	12	0.0
			Over-the-counter Medication	656	2.6
			Prescription Medication	312	1.2
			Other Nonfood Advertising	6,722	27.0
All Nonfood Products	**19,549**	**78.4**	**All Nonfood Products**	**19,549**	**78.4**
Total	24,939		Total	24,939	

Source: Staff analysis of copyrighted Nielsen Media Research/Nielsen Monitor–Plus data; four weeks projected annually.

C.3. Teens and Adults

These tables provide detailed information for teens and adults.

Table C.3. Detailed Exposure to TV Advertising By Audience Share

Younger children ages 2–5

Category	All ads		Share ≥ 20%		Share ≥ 50%	
	Ads	%	Ads	%	Ads	%
Regular Cereal	160	0.6	76	0.8	13	1.3
Highly Sugared Cereal	871	3.5	694	7.7	67	7.0
Candy	441	1.8	225	2.5	3	0.3
Desserts and Dessert Ingredients	51	0.2	22	0.2	0	0.0
Cakes, Pies and Pastries	95	0.4	75	0.8	3	0.3
Regular Gum	96	0.4	53	0.6	0	0.0
Cookies	160	0.6	101	1.1	0	0.0
Ice Cream	14	0.1	2	0.0	0	0.0
Restaurants and Fast Food	1,252	5.0	456	5.1	50	5.2
Appetizers, Snacks and Nuts	354	1.4	251	2.8	18	1.9
Crackers	101	0.4	70	0.8	0	0.0
Snack, Granola and Cereal Bars	44	0.2	10	0.1	0	0.0
Dairy Products and Substitutes	370	1.5	251	2.8	28	2.9
Regular Carbonated Beverages	127	0.5	21	0.2	0	0.0
Regular Non-carbonated Beverages	261	1.0	126	1.4	0	0.0
Prepared Entrees	203	0.8	105	1.2	5	0.6
Frozen Pizza	15	0.1	1	0.0	0	0.0
Beer, Wine and Mixers	116	0.5	2	0.0	0	0.0
Diet Carbonated Beverages	19	0.1	0	0.0	0	0.0
Diet Non-carbonated Beverages	15	0.1	0	0.0	0	0.0
Fruit Juices	51	0.2	0	0.0	0	0.0
Sugarless Gum	23	0.1	5	0.1	0	0.0
Canned Fruit	0	0.0	0	0.0	0	0.0
Raisins and Other Dried Fruit	0	0.0	0	0.0	0	0.0
Fresh Fruit	0	0.0	0	0.0	0	0.0
Vegetables and Legumes	15	0.1	0	0.0	0	0.0
Meat, Poultry and Fish	44	0.2	0	0.0	0	0.0
Bread, Rolls, Waffles and Pancakes	155	0.6	105	1.2	4	0.4
Other Food and Beverage	338	1.4	113	1.3	37	3.9
All Food Products	**5,390**	**21.6**	**2,764**	**30.8**	**227**	**23.8**
Games, Toys and Hobbies	2,092	8.4	1,710	19.0	217	22.8
Screen / Audio Entertainment	1,853	7.4	846	9.4	38	4.0

Table C.3. Continued

Category	All ads		Share ≥ 20%		Share ≥ 50%	
	Ads	%	Ads	%	Ads	%
Sporting Goods	21	0.1	11	0.1	0	0.0
Exercise Equipment	0	0.0	0	0.0	0	0.0
Promos	7,065	28.3	2,493	27.7	198	20.8
PSAs	205	0.8	82	0.9	16	1.6
Dental Supplies	240	1.0	65	0.7	46	4.8
Diets and Diet Aids	58	0.2	1	0.0	0	0.0
Footwear	99	0.4	33	0.4	0	0.0
Computer Hardware and Internet Services	215	0.9	49	0.6	0	0.0
Computer Software (Non-game)	12	0.0	0	0.0	0	0.0
Over-the-counter Medication	656	2.6	43	0.5	33	3.4
Prescription Medication	312	1.2	3	0.0	0	0.0
Other Nonfood Advertising	6,722	27.0	883	9.8	179	18.8
All Nonfood Products	**19,549**	**78.4**	**6,220**	**69.2**	**727**	**76.2**
Total	24,939		8,985		954	

Source: Staff analysis of copyrighted Nielsen Media Research/Nielsen Monitor–Plus data; four weeks projected annually.

Table C.4. Annual Exposure to TV Advertising By Product Category

Teens ages 12–17

Category	Ads	%	Detailed category	Ads	%
Cereal	492	1.6	Regular Cereal	152	0.5
			Highly Sugared Cereal	340	1.1
Desserts and Sweets	806	2.6	Candy	488	1.6
			Desserts and Dessert Ingredients	44	0.1
			Cakes, Pies and Pastries	42	0.1
			Regular Gum	106	0.3
			Cookies	106	0.3
			Ice Cream	19	0.1
Restaurants and Fast Food	1,836	5.9	Restaurants and Fast Food	1,836	5.9
Snacks	332	1.1	Appetizers, Snacks and Nuts	218	0.7
			Crackers	57	0.2
			Snack, Granola and Cereal Bars	57	0.2

Dairy Products	260	0.8	Dairy Products and Substitutes	260	0.8
Sweetened Drinks	584	1.9	Regular Carbonated Beverages	289	0.9
			Regular Non-carbonated Beverages	295	0.9
Prepared Entrees	180	0.6	Prepared Entrees	155	0.5
			Frozen Pizza	25	0.1
Other Food	1,021	3.3	Beer, Wine and Mixers	276	0.9
			Diet Carbonated Beverages	36	0.1
			Diet Non-carbonated Beverages	22	0.1
			Fruit Juices	65	0.2
			Sugarless Gum	51	0.2
			Canned Fruit	0	0.0
			Raisins and Other Dried Fruit	0	0.0
			Fresh Fruit	0	0.0
			Vegetables and Legumes	22	0.1
			Meat, Poultry and Fish	72	0.2
			Bread, Rolls, Waffles and Pancakes	94	0.3
			Other Food and Beverage	383	1.2
All Food Products	**5,512**	**17.7**	**All Food Products**	**5,512**	**17.7**
Games, Toys and Hobbies	778	2.5	Games, Toys and Hobbies	778	2.5
Screen / Audio Entertainment	2,633	8.4	Screen / Audio Entertainment	2,633	8.4
Sports and Exercise	24	0.1	Sporting Goods	23	0.1
			Exercise Equipment	1	0.0
Promos and PSAs	8,007	25.7	Promos	7,803	25.0
			PSAs	204	0.7
Other Nonfood	14,235	45.6	Dental Supplies	307	1.0
			Diets and Diet Aids	132	0.4
			Footwear	190	0.6
			Computer Hardware and Internet Services	362	1.2
			Computer Software (Non-game)	20	0.1
			Over-the-counter Medication	927	3.0
			Prescription Medication	434	1.4
			Other Nonfood Advertising	11,863	38.0
All Nonfood Products	**25,677**	**82.3**	**All Nonfood Products**	**25,677**	**82.3**
Total	31,188		Total	31,188	

Source: Staff analysis of copyrighted Nielsen Media Research/Nielsen Monitor–Plus data; four weeks projected annually.

Table C.5. Annual Exposure to TV Advertising By Product Category

Category	Ads	%	Detailed category	Ads	%
			Adults ages 18 and over		
Cereal	477	0.9	Regular Cereal	286	0.5
			Highly Sugared Cereal	191	0.4
Desserts and Sweets	754	1.4	Candy	417	0.8
			Desserts and Dessert Ingredients	85	0.2
			Cakes, Pies and Pastries	24	0.0
			Regular Gum	63	0.1
			Cookies	134	0.3
			Ice Cream	31	0.1
Restaurants and Fast Food	2,546	4.9	Restaurants and Fast Food	2,546	4.9
Snacks	356	0.7	Appetizers, Snacks and Nuts	185	0.4
			Crackers	80	0.2
			Snack, Granola and Cereal Bars	92	0.2
Dairy Products	338	0.6	Dairy Products and Substitutes	338	0.6
Sweetened Drinks	479	0.9	Regular Carbonated Beverages	223	0.4
			Regular Non-carbonated Beverages	256	0.5
Prepared Entrees	323	0.6	Prepared Entrees	267	0.5
			Frozen Pizza	55	0.1
Other Food	1,939	3.7	Beer, Wine and Mixers	412	0.8
			Diet Carbonated Beverages	61	0.1
			Diet Non-carbonated Beverages	46	0.1
			Fruit Juices	170	0.3
			Sugarless Gum	52	0.1
			Canned Fruit	0	0.0
			Raisins and Other Dried Fruit	0	0.0
			Fresh Fruit	1	0.0
			Vegetables and Legumes	56	0.1
			Meat, Poultry and Fish	161	0.3
			Bread, Rolls, Waffles and Pancakes	118	0.2
			Other Food and Beverage	863	1.6
All Food Products	**7,212**	**13.7**	**All Food Products**	**7,212**	**13.7**
Games, Toys and Hobbies	414	0.8	Games, Toys and Hobbies	414	0.8

Table C.5. Continued

Category	Ads	%	Detailed category	Ads	%
Screen / Audio Entertainment	2,323	4.4	Screen / Audio Entertainment	2,323	4.4
Sports and Exercise	47	0.1	Sporting Goods	43	0.1
			Exercise Equipment	4	0.0
Promos and PSAs	12,627	24.1	Promos	12,297	23.4
			PSAs	330	0.6
Other Nonfood	29,846	56.9	Dental Supplies	589	1.1
			Diets and Diet Aids	275	0.5
			Footwear	164	0.3
			Computer Hardware and Internet Services	676	1.3
			Computer Software (Non-game)	62	0.1
			Over-the-counter Medication	2, 126	4.1
			Prescription Medication	1,263	2.4
			Other Nonfood Advertising	24,692	47.1
All Nonfood Products	**45,257**	**86.3**	**All Nonfood Products**	**45,257**	**86.3**
Total	52,469		Total	52,469	

Source: Staff analysis of copyrighted Nielsen Media Research/Nielsen Monitor–Plus data; four weeks projected annually.

D. TIME OF CHILDREN'S VIEWING

This appendix provides more detail related to the discussion in Section 3.2.

D.1. Children 2–11

Table D.1 provides more detail on children's exposure to television advertising by time of day and by type of network.

Table D.1. Percent of Advertising Exposure By Time of Day

Children ages 2-11

Time period	Overall			Cable			Broadcast		
	Sunday	Weekdays	Saturday	Sunday	Weekdays	Saturday	Sunday	Weekdays	Saturday
12 am – 2 am	0.63	2.80	0.74	0.88	3.77	0.99	0.23	1.25	0.35
2 am – 4 am	0.33	1.66	0.40	0.51	2.45	0.61	0.04	0.39	0.05
4 am – 6 am	0.23	1.13	0.23	0.37	1.69	0.36	0.02	0.24	0.03
6 am – 8 am	0.48	3.71	0.60	0.69	4.16	0.66	0.15	2.99	0.50
8 am – 10 am	1.24	4.98	2.05	1.47	6.15	1.50	0.86	3.12	2.93
10 am – 12 pm	1.28	3.94	2.25	1.75	4.97	1.72	0.54	2.31	3.09
12 pm – 2 pm	1.21	4.66	1.45	1.43	5.22	1.75	0.86	3.76	0.99
2 pm – 4 pm	1.38	6.71	1.42	1.51	6.88	1.83	1.17	6.44	0.78
4 pm – 6 pm	1.54	8.35	1.46	1.66	8.48	1.87	1.35	8.16	0.80
6 pm – 8 pm	2.11	10.66	1.69	1.79	9.59	1.97	2.62	12.36	1.26
8 pm – 10 pm	2.87	15.07	2.23	1.65	9.33	1.91	4.81	24.23	2.76
10 pm – 12 am	1.19	6.00	1.30	1.09	6.12	1.24	1.36	5.81	1.39
Daily total	14.49	69.68	15.83	14.79	68.81	16.40	14.02	71.05	14.93
Weekly exposure (ads per child)		491			302			190	

Source: Staff analysis of copyrighted Nielsen Media Research/Nielsen Monitor-Plus data; four weeks projected annually.

In Section 3.4 we looked at how children's exposure to product ads varies over different types of shows, where shows are grouped by the share of children in the audience. Looking at shows based on the number of children watching provides additional insight. We group the shows based on the number of children watching — or the percentage of the population of children that watch the show. We consider (in addition to exposure on all shows) exposure on shows with at least 1.0 percent and at least 3.0 percent of children watching; or, approximately, shows with at least 394,800 children watching and shows with at least 1,184,400 children watching.[73] Only 4.5 percent of all ads are aired on shows that are watched by more than one percent of children. However, 51 percent of children's ad exposure is from shows in which one percent or more of children are watching. Only 0.9 percent of all ads are aired on shows that are watched by more than three percent of children. However, 19 percent of children's ad exposure is from these shows.[74]

This appendix presents results of this analysis for all children and for younger children.

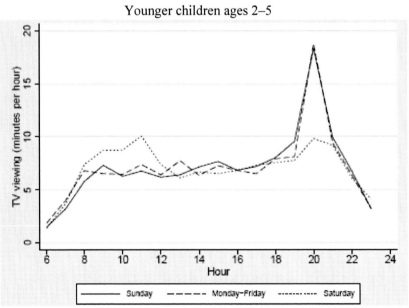

Source: Staff analysis of copyrighted Nielsen Media Research/Nielsen Monitor–Plus data; four weeks projected annually.

Figure D.1. TV Viewing Over the Day.

Younger children ages 2–5

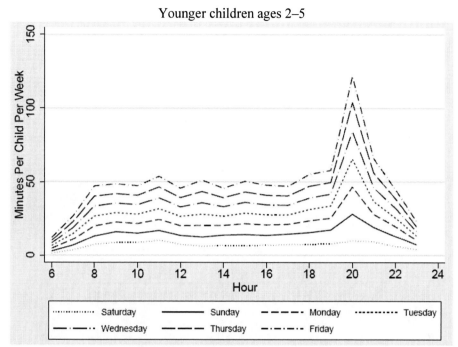

Figure D.2. Cumulative TV Viewing Per Hour over the Week.

D.2. YOUNGER CHILDREN 2–5

This section provides information for younger children comparable to that presented for all children in Section 3.2. In addition, as for all children above, we present a table with more detail on younger children's exposure to television advertising by time of day and by type of network.

Younger children ages 2–5, cable (a) and broadcast (b)

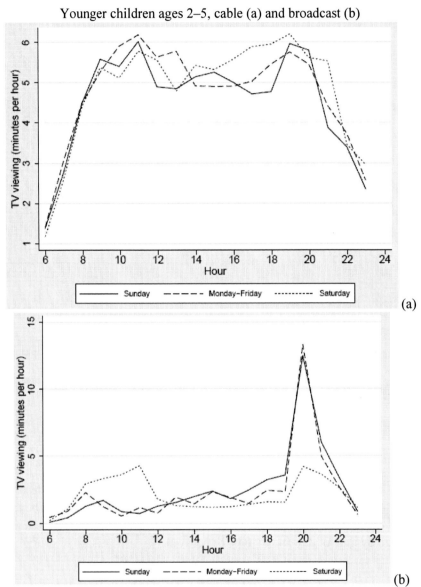

(a)

(b)

Source: Staff analysis of copyrighted Nielsen Media Research/Nielsen Monitor–Plus data;
    four weeks projected annually.
Note: Graphs on different scales.

Figure D.3. TV Viewing Over the Day.

Younger children ages 2–5

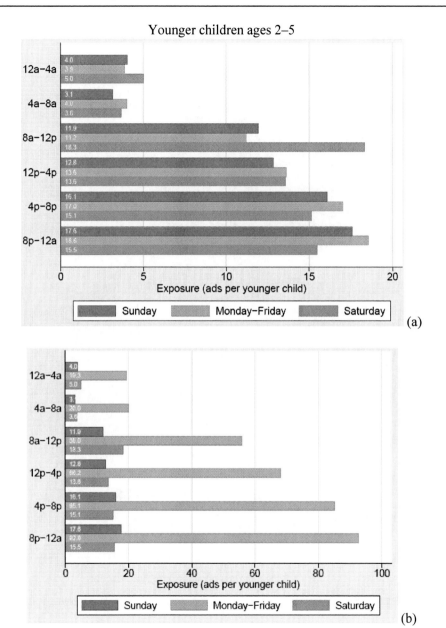

(a)

(b)

Source: Staff analysis of copyrighted Nielsen Media Research/Nielsen Monitor–Plus data;
   four weeks projected annually.
Note: Graphs on different scales.

Figure D.4. Average (a) and Total (b) Exposure to TV Advertising over the Day.

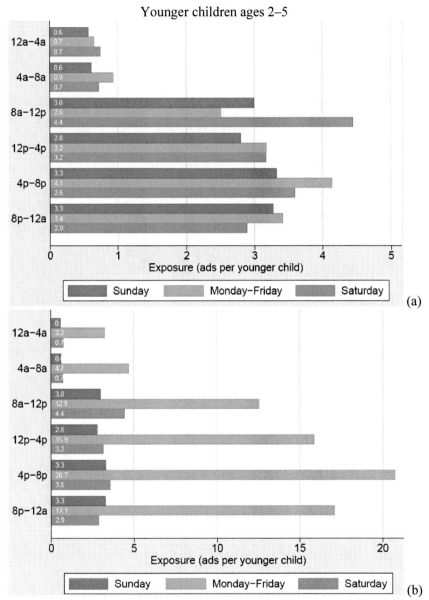

(a)

(b)

Source: Staff analysis of copyrighted Nielsen Media Research/Nielsen Monitor–Plus data;
    four weeks projected annually.
Note: Graphs on different scales.

Figure D.5. Average (a) and Total (b) Exposure to Food Advertising over the Day.

Younger children ages 2–5

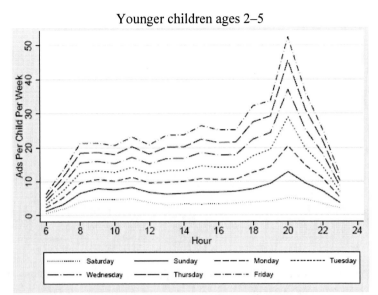

Source: Staff analysis of copyrighted Nielsen Media Research/Nielsen Monitor–Plus data; four weeks projected annually.

Figure D.6. Cumulative Exposure to TV Advertising Per Hour over the Week.

Younger children ages 2–5, cable (a) and broadcast (b)

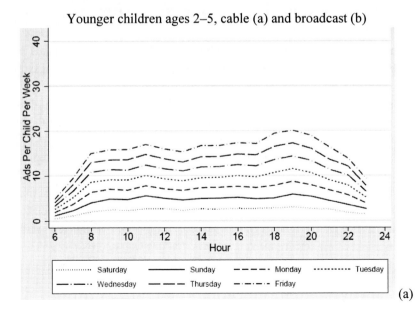

(a)

Figure D.7. (Continued)

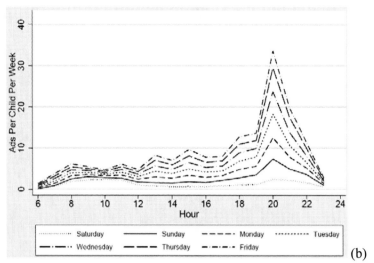

(b)

Source: Staff analysis of copyrighted Nielsen Media Research/Nielsen Monitor–Plus data;
four weeks projected annually.

Figure D.7. Cumulative Exposure to TV Advertising Per Hour over the Week.

E. EXPOSURE BY SIZE OF CHILD AUDIENCE

In Section 3.4 we looked at how children's exposure to product ads varies over different types of shows, where shows are grouped by the share of children in the audience. Looking at shows based on the number of children watching provides additional insight. We group the shows based on the number of children watching — or the percentage of the population of children that watch the show. We consider (in addition to exposure on all shows) exposure on shows with at least 1.0 percent and at least 3.0 percent of children watching; or, approximately, shows with at least 394,800 children watching and shows with at least 1,184,400 children watching.[73] Only 4.5 percent of all ads are aired on shows that are watched by more than one percent of children. However, 51 percent of children's ad exposure is from shows in which one percent or more of children are watching. Only 0.9 percent of all ads are aired on shows that are watched by more than three percent of children. However, 19 percent of children's ad exposure is from these shows.[74]

This appendix presents results of this analysis for all children and for younger children.

Table D.2. Percent of Advertising Exposure by Time of Day

Younger children ages 2-5

Time period	Overall			Cable			Broadcast		
	Sunday	Weekdays	Saturday	Sunday	Weekdays	Saturday	Sunday	Weekdays	Saturday
12 am – 2 am	0.56	2.51	0.67	0.73	3.31	0.87	0.25	1.09	0.31
2 am – 4 am	0.28	1.53	0.38	0.42	2.19	0.56	0.03	0.34	0.04
4 am – 6 am	0.23	1.05	0.24	0.34	1.52	0.35	0.01	0.21	0.02
6 am – 8 am	0.43	3.13	0.53	0.59	3.54	0.56	0.14	2.41	0.46
8 am – 10 am	1.20	5.88	1.81	1.41	7.14	1.49	0.83	3.63	2.40
10 am – 12 pm	1.29	5.84	2.02	1.72	7.34	1.65	0.53	3.15	2.67
12 pm – 2 pm	1.28	6.56	1.45	1.49	7.05	1.66	0.91	5.68	1.06
2 pm – 4 pm	1.40	7.69	1.39	1.54	7.64	1.72	1.16	7.78	0.81
4 pm – 6 pm	1.45	7.62	1.46	1.49	7.95	1.80	1.39	7.03	0.86
6 pm – 8 pm	1.90	10.18	1.70	1.65	9.31	1.92	2.36	11.75	1.30
8 pm – 10 pm	2.58	13.87	2.07	1.49	8.27	1.73	4.54	23.91	2.68
10 pm – 12 am	1.10	5.53	1.16	0.93	5.51	1.10	1.39	5.57	1.27
Daily total	13.72	71.40	14.88	13.81	70.77	15.42	13.55	72.54	13.91
Weekly exposure (ads per younger child)		478			307			171	

Source: Staff analysis of copyrighted Nielsen Media Research/Nielsen Monitor-Plus data; four weeks projected annually.

Table E.1. Annual Exposure to TV Advertising By Child Audience Size

Children ages 2–11

Category	All ads		GRP ≥ 1.0		GRP ≥ 3.0	
	Ads	%	Ads	%	Ads	%
Cereal	993	3.9	816	6.3	365	7.7
Desserts and Sweets	898	3.5	613	4.7	225	4.7
Restaurants and Fast Food	1, 367	5.3	823	6.3	281	5.9
Snacks	490	1.9	366	2.8	148	3.1
Dairy Products	353	1.4	259	2.0	123	2.6
Sweetened Drinks	430	1.7	252	1.9	117	2.5
Prepared Entrees	222	0.9	143	1.1	55	1.2
Other Food	786	3.1	340	2.6	140	3.0
All Food Products	**5, 538**	**21.6**	**3,612**	**27.7**	**1,454**	**30.7**
Games, Toys and Hobbies	1, 909	7.5	1, 727	13.2	726	15.3
Screen / Audio Entertainment	2, 010	7.8	1, 330	10.2	576	12.2
Sports and Exercise	24	0.1	13	0.1	7	0.1
Promos and PSAs	7, 305	28.5	3, 360	25.8	1, 054	22.3
Other Nonfood	8, 842	34.5	3, 002	23.0	916	19.4
All Nonfood Products	**20, 091**	**78.4**	**9,432**	**72.3**	**3, 279**	**69.3**
Total	25,629		13,044		4,733	

Source: Staff analysis of copyrighted Nielsen Media Research/Nielsen Monitor–Plus data; four weeks projected annually.

Table E.2. Annual Exposure to TV Advertising By Audience Size

Younger children ages 2–5

Category	All ads		GRP ≥ 1.0		GRP ≥ 3.0	
	Ads	%	Ads	%	Ads	%
Cereal	1,031	4.1	836	6.5	470	8.3
Desserts and Sweets	857	3.4	575	4.5	228	4.0
Restaurants and Fast Food	1,252	5.0	760	5.9	314	5.6
Snacks	499	2.0	373	2.9	181	3.2
Dairy Products	370	1.5	275	2.1	157	2.8
Sweetened Drinks	388	1.6	231	1.8	103	1.8
Prepared Entrees	218	0.9	138	1.1	64	1.1
Other Food	776	3.1	349	2.7	187	3.3

All Food Products	5,390	21.6	3,535	27.6	1,705	30.2
Games, Toys and Hobbies	2,092	8.4	1,888	14.7	1,084	19.2
Screen / Audio Entertainment	1,853	7.4	1,234	9.6	570	10.1
Sports and Exercise	21	0.1	12	0.1	6	0.1
Promos and PSAs	7,270	29.2	3,273	25.6	1,212	21.5
Other Nonfood	8,314	33.3	2,866	22.4	1,061	18.8
All Nonfood Products	19,549	78.4	9,273	72.4	3,933	69.8
Total	24,939		12,809		5,638	

Source: Staff analysis of copyrighted Nielsen Media Research/Nielsen Monitor–Plus data; four weeks projected annually.

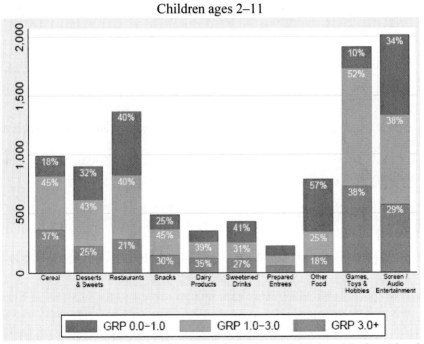

Source: Staff analysis of copyrighted Nielsen Media Research/Nielsen Monitor–Plus data; four weeks projected annually.

Figure E.1. Annual Exposure to TV Advertising By Child Audience Size, Selected Categories.

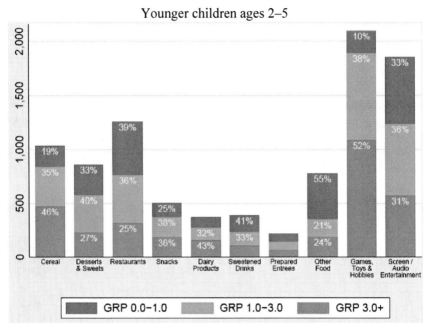

Source: Staff analysis of copyrighted Nielsen Media Research/Nielsen Monitor{Plus data; four weeks projected annually.

Note: Promos and PSAs and Other Nonfood Advertising omitted because they dominate the graph.

Figure E.2. Annual Exposure to TV Advertising By Audience Size.

F. HOW SIZE AND SHARE OF AUDIENCE ARE RELATED

This appendix provides more information related to the analysis in Section 3.5. We present a table similar to Table 3.7, except we show how ads aired vary by GRP and share alongside the analysis of exposure to ads. For younger children, we present tables comparable to those for all children in Section 3.5 as well as a table analyzing both ads aired and exposure to ads.

Table F.1. Percent of Ads Aired and Exposure by Audience Size (GRP) and Audience Share

Children ages 2–11

ALL ADS

Total ads aired   13,395,154   Total exposure   25,629

GRP	0–20	Share 20–50	≥ 50	Total		GRP	0–20	Share 20–50	≥ 50	Total
0.0 – 1.0	91.4	2.7	1.5	95.7		0.0 – 1.0	41.2	5.3	2.5	49.1
1.0 – 3.0	1.0	0.7	1.7	3.4		1.0 – 3.0	8.6	5.9	17.9	32.4
≥ 3.0	0.1	0.1	0.6	0.8		≥ 3.0	3.2	1.9	13.4	18.5
Total	92.6	3.5	3.9	100.0		Total	53.0	13.1	33.8	100.0

ADS ON CABLE

% ads aired   82.6   % exposure   61.4

GRP	0–20	Share 20–50	≥ 50	Total		GRP	0–20	Share 20–50	≥ 50	Total
0.0 – 1.0	92.4	2.5	1.8	96.7		0.0 – 1.0	35.5	6.1	3.9	45.5
1.0 – 3.0	0.0	0.5	2.0	2.6		1.0 – 3.0	0.3	5.2	28.7	34.2
≥ 3.0	0.0	0.0	0.7	0.7		≥ 3.0	0.0	0.0	20.3	20.3
Total	92.4	3.0	4.5	100.0		Total	35.8	11.3	52.9	100.0

ADS ON BROADCAST

% ads aired   17.3   % exposure   38.6

GRP	0–20	Share 20–50	≥ 50	Total		GRP	0–20	Share 20–50	≥ 50	Total
0.0 – 1.0	86.9	3.9	0.4	91.2		0.0 – 1.0	50.4	4.2	0.3	54.9
1.0 – 3.0	5.9	1.6	0.2	7.6		1.0 – 3.0	21.8	7.0	0.9	29.6
≥ 3.0	0.7	0.3	0.1	1.2		≥ 3.0	8.3	4.9	2.3	15.5
Total	93.5	5.8	0.7	100.0		Total	80.4	16.1	3.5	100.0

Source: Staff analysis of copyrighted Nielsen Media Research/Nielsen Monitor–Plus data; four weeks projected annually.

G. SEASONAL PATTERNS IN ADVERTISING EXPOSURE

These tables illustrate the seasonal variation in children's exposure to advertising. The major difference is that exposure to food advertising is much lower in November than other months, displaced primarily by Games, Toys and

Hobbies and to a lesser extent by Screen/Audio Entertainment. Overall exposure to advertising is highest in November and lowest in the summer (May for children and July for younger children).

Table F.2. Percent of Ad Exposure By Audience Size (GRP) and Audience Share

Younger children ages 25

All adS   24,939 ads

GRP		Share			Total
		020	2050	> 50	
0.0	1.0	45.3	3.3	0.1	48.6
1.0	3.0	15.0	13.8	0.0	28.8
>3.0		3.8	15.1	3.7	22.6
Total		64.0	32.2	3.8	100.0

Ads on cable   64.2% exposure

GRP	Share			Total
	0–20	20–50	> 50	
0.0 – 1.0	38.2	4.9	0.1	43.2
1.0 – 3.0	7.3	20.9	0.0	28.2
>3.0	0.3	22.6	5.7	28.6
Total	45.8	48.4	5.8	100.0

Ads on broadcast   35.8% exposure

GRP	Share			Total
	0–20	20–50	> 50	
0.0 – 1.0	57.8	0.5	0.0	58.3
1.03.0	28.7	1.1	0.1	29.8
>3.0	10.0	1.7	0.2	11.9
Total	96.5	3.2	0.3	100.0

Source: Staff analysis of copyrighted Nielsen Media Research/Nielsen Monitor–Plus data; four weeks projected annually.

Table F.3. Percent of Food Ad Exposure By Audience Size (GRP) and Audience

Share Younger children ages 25

All ads   5,390 ads

		Share			
GRP		020	2050	> 50	Total
0.0	1.0	30.8	3.5	0.1	34.4
1.0	3.0	14.6	19.3	0.0	34.0
>3.0		3.2	24.3	4.1	31.6
Total		48.7	47.1	4.2	100.0

AdS On Cable   75.3% exposure

	Share			
GRP	0–20	20–50	> 50	Total
0.0 – 1.0	24.3	4.5	0.1	29.0
1.0 – 3.0	8.4	25.2	0.0	33.6
>3.0	0.5	31.5	5.4	37.4
Total	33.3	61.2	5.5	100.0

Ads on broadcast   24.7% exposure

	Share			
GRP	0–20	20–50	> 50	Total
0.0 – 1.0	50.7	0.3	0.0	51.0
1.03.0	33.6	1.4	0.1	35.1
>3.0	11.4	2.3	0.2	13.9
Total	95.8	3.9	0.3	100.0

Source: Staff analysis of copyrighted Nielsen Media Research/Nielsen Monitor–Plus data; four weeks projected annually.

Table F.4. Percent of Ads Aired and Exposure by Audience Size (GRP) and Audience Share

Children ages 2–5 All adS

ALL ADS

| Total ads aired | | | | 13,395,154 | Total exposure | | | | 24,939 |

GRP	Share 0–20	20–50	≥ 50	Total	GRP	Share 0–20	20–50	≥ 50	Total
0.0 – 1.0	94.3	1.7	0.0	96.0	0.0 – 1.0	45.3	3.3	0.1	48.6
1.0 – 3.0	1.8	1.2	0.0	3.0	1.0 – 3.0	15.0	13.8	0.0	28.8
≥ 3.0	0.1	0.7	0.1	1.0	≥ 3.0	3.8	15.1	3.7	22.6
Total	96.3	3.6	0.2	100.0	Total	64.0	32.2	3.8	100.0

ADS ON CABLE

| % ads aired | | | | 82.6 | % exposure | | | | 64.2 |

GRP	Share 0–20	20–50	≥ 50	Total	GRP	Share 0–20	20–50	≥ 50	Total
0.0 – 1.0	94.9	1.9	0.0	96.9	0.0 – 1.0	38.2	4.9	0.1	43.2
1.0 – 3.0	0.7	1.4	0.0	2.1	1.0 – 3.0	7.3	20.9	0.0	28.2
≥ 3.0	0.0	0.8	0.2	1.0	≥ 3.0	0.3	22.6	5.7	28.6
Total	95.6	4.2	0.2	100.0	Total	45.8	48.4	5.8	100.0

ADS ON BROADCAST

| % ads aired | | | | 17.3 | % exposure | | | | 35.8 |

GRP	Share 0–20	20–50	≥ 50	Total	GRP	Share 0–20	20–50	≥ 50	Total
0.0 – 1.0	91.6	0.4	0.0	92.0	0.0 – 1.0	57.8	0.5	0.0	58.3
1.0 – 3.0	7.0	0.2	0.0	7.2	1.0 – 3.0	28.7	1.1	0.1	29.8
≥ 3.0	0.8	0.1	0.0	0.9	≥ 3.0	10.0	1.7	0.2	11.9
Total	99.3	0.6	0.0	100.0	Total	96.5	3.2	0.3	100.0

Source: Staff analysis of copyrighted Nielsen Media Research/Nielsen Monitor–Plus data; four weeks projected annually.

Table G.1. Annual Exposure to Advertising Computed From Each Month

Children ages 2–11

Category	November		February		May		July	
	Ads	%	Ads	%	Ads	%	Ads	%
Cereal	563	2.1	1,193	4.6	1,056	4.4	1,159	4.6
Desserts and Sweets	316	1.2	1, 140	4.4	1, 101	4.6	1,035	4.1
Restaurants and Fast Food	1,138	4.1	1,430	5.5	1,328	5.6	1,572	6.2

Category	Ads	%	Ads	%	Ads	%	Ads	%
Snacks	148	0.5	667	2.6	705	3.0	439	1.7
Dairy Products	220	0.8	426	1.6	562	2.4	206	0.8
Sweetened Drinks	127	0.5	362	1.4	659	2.8	573	2.3
Prepared Entrees	175	0.6	334	1.3	123	0.5	255	1.0
Other Food	696	2.5	760	2.9	749	3.1	940	3.7
All Food Products	**3,382**	**12.3**	**6,311**	**24.2**	**6,282**	**26.4**	**6,178**	**24.5**
Games, Toys and Hobbies	5,732	20.9	1,073	4.1	613	2.6	220	0.9
Screen / Audio Entertainment	2,787	10.2	1,559	6.0	1,707	7.2	1,988	7.9
Sports and Exercise	9	0.0	9	0.0	35	0.1	42	0.2
Promos and PSAs	7,271	26.5	7,428	28.4	6,673	28.0	7,850	31.2
Other Nonfood	8,235	30.0	9,735	37.3	8,482	35.7	8,916	35.4
All Nonfood Products	**24,035**	**87.7**	**19,803**	**75.8**	**17,510**	**73.6**	**19,015**	**75.5**
Total	27,417		26,114		23,792		25,193	

Source: Staff analysis of copyrighted Nielsen Media Research/Nielsen Monitor–Plus data; four weeks projected annually.

Table G.2. Annual Exposure to Advertising Computed From Each Month

Category	November		February		May		July	
	Ads	%	Ads	%	Ads	%	Ads	%
Cereal	616	2.2	1,233	4.8	1,203	5.1	1,072	4.8
Desserts and Sweets	319	1.1	1,111	4.3	1,104	4.7	893	4.0
Restaurants and Fast Food	1,069	3.8	1,369	5.4	1,228	5.2	1,340	6.0
Snacks	157	0.6	685	2.7	757	3.2	396	1.8
Dairy Products	219	0.8	448	1.8	624	2.6	190	0.9
Sweetened Drinks	120	0.4	333	1.3	633	2.7	467	2.1
Prepared Entrees	181	0.6	338	1.3	124	0.5	230	1.0
Other Food	690	2.4	781	3.1	754	3.2	877	3.9
All Food Products	**3,372**	**11.9**	**6,297**	**24.6**	**6,426**	**27.3**	**5,463**	**24.5**
Games, Toys and Hobbies	6,441	22.8	1,113	4.3	618	2.6	195	0.9
Screen / Audio Entertainment	2,768	9.8	1,438	5.6	1,600	6.8	1,605	7.2
Sports and Exercise	7	0.0	8	0.0	33	0.1	37	0.2
Promos and PSAs	7,647	27.0	7,422	29.0	6,838	29.0	7,172	32.2
Other Nonfood	8,064	28.5	9,305	36.4	8,059	34.2	7,826	35.1
All Nonfood Products	**24,927**	**88.1**	**19,285**	**75.4**	**17,149**	**72.7**	**16,835**	**75.5**
Total	28,299		25,582		23,575		22,299	

Source: Staff analysis of copyrighted Nielsen Media Research/Nielsen Monitor–Plus data; four weeks projected annually.

ACKNOWLEDGEMENTS

We would like to thank our FTC colleagues as well as workshop and conference participants for their useful comments on our preliminary findings. Alexi Charter, Brian Murphy, and Michael Lovinger provided valuable research assistance.

ENDNOTES

[1.] *Federal Register* / Vol. 72, No. 74 / Wednesday, April 18, 2007 / Notices. See also Moore (2006) on advergaming.

[2.] See Gantz et al. (2007) for a recent content analysis of television advertising on children's and general interest programming. Neither this report nor Gantz et al. (2007) considers whether children may respond differently to the types of ads aired on children's programs.

[3.] The FTC is beginning a study to attempt to gauge the extent of these other forms of marketing to children. Federal Register / Vol. 72, No. 74 / Wednesday, April 18, 2007 / Notices.

[4.] Promotions are ads for other television shows or networks and will often be referred to as 'Promos' in this report. Screen/Audio Entertainment includes ads for movies, computer games, video games, DVDs and CDs.

[5.] 96 percent of all ads aired had a children's viewership of less than one percent of the child population. Approximately half of their ad exposure comes from these shows.

[6.] None of the shows in our data had a child audience larger than 10 percent of the child population. Very few had a child audience greater than five percent of the child population. Only 19 percent of children's ad exposure came from shows with a child audience greater than three percent of the child population.

[7.] In 2004 children were 14.3 percent of the population of those two and older – the potential viewing audience.

[8.] According to the CAB, cable attracted about 33 percent of television advertising dollars in the fourth quarter of 2003 and 36 percent in the fourth quarter of 2004 Cabletelevision Advertising Bureau (2006e).

[9.] See Television Bureau of Advertising (2006a), which is based on data from the first quarter of 2006.

[10.] TV viewing in 1977 from A. C. Nielsen Co. (1977); in 2004, ad-supported figure from staff analysis of Nielsen data. Total 2004 children's figure from

Television Bureau of Advertising (2006b). Teens' television watching also declined but not as steeply as children's.

[11.] See Appendix A for a detailed description of the data and methods we used in our analysis.

[12.] For brevity, we will refer to the 2003–2004 programming season as 2004.

[13.] Gantz et al. (2007) examined sponsorship messages on Disney and PBS along with standard advertising; they found a very limited number of ad-like sponsorship messages, less than half of which related to food. However, the omission of these networks and pay cable networks from our data clearly causes an underestimate of exposure to Promotions.

[14.] National advertising refers to advertising purchased from national networks or through national syndication that airs nationally. In contrast, local spot (spot) advertising is purchased from a single station and airs only on that station.

[15.] 15A children's GRP of 2 means that 2 percent of the 2–11 population is estimated to be watching a given program.

[16.] Note we first multiplied each ad's GRP by the population and then divided by the population again at the end. Equivalently, one can calculate the day's exposure by just summing the GRPs (and dividing by 100 since GRPs are expressed as whole numbers rather than percents).

[17.] From here on we will focus attention to children 2-11, teens 12-17, and adults. The appendices include analogous results for younger children 2-5.

[18.] The average is 25.1 for children and 25.5 for adults.

[19.] Our estimates differ from other published estimates of children's exposure to television advertising; a widely cited estimate is more than 50 percent higher than ours (Kunkel and Gantz 1992). Why are these estimates so far apart? First, we have more detailed data than other researchers have used over the past three decades. Most researchers have relied on aggregate estimates of the amount of time that children watch television each day, combined with counts of ads aired per hour on selected samples of TV programming. These methods can be accurate so long as the component pieces are accurate representations of children's viewing habits. For example, in our 2004 data, an average of 30 ads were aired per hour and children watched an average of 2.3 hours of ad-supported television per day. A "back of the envelope" calculation yields an estimate that children saw 25,185 ads per year, which compares quite well with our direct GRP estimate. ($30 \times 2.3 \times 365 = 25,185$) See Section 6.3 for a further discussion of research implications.

[20.] According to Kimmelman (2004), the "top 10 cable networks account for 50 percent of all viewing, and the top 20 channels account for 75 percent of all viewing." Our Nielsen data includes 50 ad-supported cable networks, 7 broadcast networks, and nationally syndicated programming.

21. See Appendix A for a detailed description of our method.

22. There are more sources of television programming presented without advertisements now than in 1977. Numerous cable channels as well as public television channels are not supported by advertising. We estimate that in 2004, viewing of ad-supported television accounted for about 70 percent of children's overall TV viewing. Nielsen analysis of television viewing in 2006 finds that around 73 percent of children's viewing was on ad-supported programming a difference of about 5 minutes per day from our 2004 estimate based on 4 weeks of data. In 1977, ad-free programming was generally limited to, at most, one public television channel per market.

23. We find an average of about 30 ads aired per hour in our data. The frequency of ads on shows with the largest child (and adult) audiences is, unsurprisingly, higher than on the average show aired. Accounting for viewing habits, we find that children on average see about 31 ads per hour (22.0 paid ads per hour), teenagers see about 34 ads per hour, and adults see about 35 ads per hour.

24. There are also changes in children's exposure to advertising over the seasons; they see fewer food ads in November, for example. See Appendix G for details.

25. Appendix A discusses the choice of product categories. Appendix B describes how we define each of our categories. In most cases, that simply involves associating one or more product category codes in the Nielsen data with one of our categories. In some cases, our categories include only part of a Nielsen product category. For example, our juice category includes only 100 percent juice while the juice product category code includes juice drinks that are not pure juice.

26. The remainder of the results in the body of the report are presented in terms of the broader categories. Appendix C presents more results at the detailed level.

27. These two categories are now in Other Nonfood Advertising.

28. The Games, Toys, and Hobbies category does have a few items that are not sedentary — small riding toys, for instance. But most of the items are associated with relatively quiet, if not completely sedentary, pastimes. Bicycles and skateboards are not included; they are in Sports and Exercise.

29. More precisely, we are grouping ads based on the share of children in the audience of a particular episode at the time the ad was aired.

30. We also looked at how exposure to different product categories changed as the child audience size changed. We found little in the way of systematic patterns. That analysis is described in Appendix E.

31. Note our use of the term is different than the industry standard. "Share" is generally used to refer to the percent of people watching television who are tuned to a given show.

32. In some tables and figures, we examine ad exposure on shows with a child share between 20 and 50 percent and refer to that grouping as family shows as well. Labels will clearly indicate whether we are talking about the 20 to 50 percent range or all shows with a child share greater than 20 percent.

33. All figures omit Sports and Exercise, Promos and PSAs, and Other Nonfood. Exposure to advertising in the Sports and Exercise category is such a small percentage of total exposure that it would be barely visible in graphs. Exposure to advertising in both Promos and PSAs and Other Nonfood is more than three times as large as any other category; their inclusion would alter the scale and obscure differences in other categories of interest.

34. Appendix F gives more information on the relationship between size and share.

35. Because of their smaller proportion in the population, it is, of course, more difficult for younger children to constitute 50 percent of any audience. Children 2–5 are 5.6 percent of the two and over U.S. population; children 2–11 are 14.3 percent of the two and over U.S. population.

36. 36A complete list of PCC codes assigned to this category can be found in Appendix B.

37. The concern at that time was television advertising of food products that contribute to tooth decay.

38. At the time of this report, there were no detailed studies on how much of children's viewing time was devoted to network programs. The Economist (1981) reports that, in 1975, 93 percent of television viewing was captured by network affiliates. According to Adler, networks supplied approximately 70 percent of their affiliates programming. (The remainder was either locally produced or syndicated programming.) Another study, discussed below, analyzed exposure to spot ads. Spot ads include all ads on non-network shows as well as local or regional ads aired during network programs. Approximately two-thirds of available ad time during network programs (in the late 1970s) was taken by network supplied advertising; the remaining was available for station identification, public service announcements, and local or regional advertising.

39. The results reported in this section are based on Abel's Tables XVI through XXI (pp. 64-70). Those Tables report estimated Gross Impressions for children 2-11 in each of the product categories. "Gross impressions" are defined by Abel as "an estimate of the probable number of exposures for advertising messages. It is obtained by multiplying the number of 30-second advertisements for a brand product by the audience for the program in which the advertisement appeared. In this study, these gross impressions were then summed across all brand products within a product category" (62) We convert gross impressions into an exposure measure comparable to that used in analyzing the 2004 data. Exposures are gross impressions divided by the child population figures from Abel's Appendix B and multiplied by 100. Exposures are annualized by multiplying by 365/89 where 89 is the number of days in his three months of data.

40. Children 2-11 were 16.5 percent of the potential viewing audience — the population of those two and over.

41. There were 46 shows with at least a 20 percent child audience share in February, 44 in May, and 41 in November.

42. There were 40 shows with at least 3.5 million children in the audience in February, 16 in May, and 27 in November.

43. The results reported in this section are based on Table 1 (page 5), Table B-3 (page 46), Table B-6 (page 49), and Table B-9 (page 52) from Beales' report. The audience was measured by gross impressions, which Beales defined as the minutes of advertising times the number of people in the audience. According to Arbitron Television estimates, there were 159,928,100 persons two years old and older in television households in these 75 markets, and 24,798,200 children 2–11, in 1977. Thus, children were 15.51 percent of the potential audience in these cities (Beales 1978, vi). We convert gross impressions into an exposure measure comparable to that used in analyzing the 2004 data. Exposures are gross impressions divided by the child population figures above and multiplied by 100. We then divide by 2 to get exposure to ads instead of minutes (Abel's definition of gross impression was based on 30 seconds, which was the length of nearly all ads in 1977). Exposures are annualized by multiplying by 365/28 where 28 is the number of days in his four weeks of data.

44. Audience estimates were not available for some of the dayparts in each of the months; these dayparts were excluded from the analysis. According to Beales, advertising in those dayparts accounted for approximately 16 percent of total advertising minutes. Therefore, his estimates understate exposure to spot

advertising. We do not know whether advertising in the omitted dayparts had a product mix similar to those analyzed.

[45.] The Adler et al. (1977) estimate is consistent with other publicly available information from the period. For example, according to Economist (1981), network affiliates accounted for 93 percent of all TV viewing in 1975. Suppose this also held in 1977. In 1977, networks supplied about 70 percent of affiliates' programming and about two-thirds of ads on network programming (Abel 1978). These figures, combined with Beales' non-network exposure estimate implies children saw, on average, 21,948 ads.

[46.] 46A very high percentage of ads in 1977 were 30 seconds long; Adler et al. (1977, citing Barcus (1975)), reports that 98 percent of commercials monitored in his studies were 30 seconds in length. In 2004, the average television ad is 25 seconds long.

[47.] Abel also analyzed shows watched by at least 3.5 million children. However, in assessing children's food ad exposure in 1977 we will focus on his sample selected by the child audience share.

[48.] Jn our 2004 data, Promos and PSAs make up a similar fraction of ad exposure on all types of programming.

[49.] We estimate Promos and PSAs to be in Abel's network shows by 2,735/0.9 - 2, 735 = 304, and in Beales' dayparts by 11, 194/0.9 - 11, 194 = 1,244. Then the new estimated totals for Abel and Beales are 2,735+304 = 3,039 and 11, 194 + 1,244 = 12, 438. We subtract these Abel and Beales totals from the NSF (Adler) estimates to find the exposure missing from Abel's network study, 21, 904 - 3,039 - 12,438 = 6,427.

[50.] That is, $(32.6 - 22.6)/32.6 = 0.307$.

[51.] That is, $(1 - .307) \times 61.9 = 42.9$.

[52.] This estimate parallels standard industry data on ad expenditures which shows that 26.4 percent of national TV ad spending was for food in 1977. In 2004, food ad spending on national TV had dropped to 17.1 percent (BAR/LNA 1977, 2004).

[53.] That is, applying this ratio to Abel's estimate of the percent of expenditures that are food, shown in Table 5.4, we get 1:36 x 24:4 = 33:2.

[54.] That is, from Table 5.2 we know that children saw 9,466 national ads (6,427 + 3,039). Thus children's exposure to national food ads would be $0.332 \times 9,466 = 3, 143$.

[55.] For comparison, we present the calculation based on the other approach. As discussed above, Table 5.3 suggests the percentage of food ads on all national shows in 1977 was 42.9 percent. Thus children's exposure to national food ads would be 0.429 × (6,427 + 3,039) = 4,061 and overall exposure to food ads would be 4,061 + 2,941 = 7,002.

[56.] The other approach finds a decline of about 21 percent. ((7,002 - 5, 538)/7, 002 = 0.21)

[57.] For children's food ad exposure in 2004 to be at the same level as in 1977, children would have to have seen 2,597 national network food ads in 1977 (that is, 5,538 (2004 level) - 2,941 (Beales 1977), or 27.4 percent of their national ad exposure (that is, 2, 597/(6, 427 + 3,039) = 27.4%.

[58.] Moreover, note that if we suppose there were no food advertisements at all on any of the programs with a child audience share less than 20 percent we can determine an absolute upper limit on any potential increase in children's food ad exposure. In that case, children would have seen 4,520 food ads in 1977 (the sum of the Abel and Beales estimates), compared to 5,538 food ads in 2004, a 23 percent increase. Obviously, this is an unreasonable scenario, because food was advertised on general audience shows in 1977, but it sets an absolute upper limit on how much food advertising could have increased, and it requires a clearly unreasonable assumption to get to that level.

[59.] Biskind (1998): "But cThe Godfather's' advertising strategy was traditional: ads in newspapers. In those days, producers sometimes bought local TV time to promote regional openings of B movies, but nobody bought network time .... Besides TV was regarded as a rival medium."

[60.] Computer games, video games, computer toys, and entertainment software.

[61.] We also find that 56% of children's exposure to all cable advertising and 70% of children's exposure to food advertising on cable comes from two cable networks.

[62.] See Gantz et al. (2007) for a recent content analysis of television advertising on children's and general interest programming. Neither this report nor Gantz et al. (2007) considers whether children may respond differently to the types of ads aired on children's programs.

[63.] See, for example, CSPI (2003), Hastings et al. (2003), IOM (2005), Rideout and Hamel (2006).

[64.] See Table 3.8.

[65.] The FTC is beginning a study to attempt to gauge the extent of these other forms of marketing to children. Federal Register / Vol. 72, No. 74 / Wednesday, April 18, 2007 / Notices.

[66.] These shows do, however, contain promotions for other programming.

[67.] The data cover 9 national English- and Spanish-language broadcast networks (ABC, CBS, FOX, NBC, Telefutura, Telemundo, UPN, Univision, and WB) and 50 national cable networks. UPN and WB have since merged to form the CW network.

[68.] These 75 metropolitan areas include 78.6 percent of the U.S. population.

[69.] Staff collected nutritional information from the Internet and in person during the summer of 2005. (The National Nutrient Database for Standard Reference can be found at http://www.ars.usda.gov/main/site_ main. htm?modecode =12-35-45- 00, last visited April 12, 2007.)

[70.] Appendix B presents a detailed list of which PCCs and brand categories were assigned to each study category.

[71.] Note this is equivalent to simply summing the GRPs; however, there are programming advantages to following the two-step procedure.

[72.] 239 PCCs were assigned to Other Nonfood.

[73.] These numbers are calculated based on Nielsen-provided population figures for 2-11 year-olds for the fall of 2003.

[74.] We find that nearly 93 percent of all television episodes are watched by fewer than one percent of children.

REFERENCES

A. C. Nielsen Co. 1977. Television Audience: 1977. Media Research Services Group.

Abel, John D. 1978. The Child Audience for Network Television Programming and Advertising. Children's Advertising Rulemaking Comment, Submitted to the Federal Trade Comission.

Adler, Richard P., B Friedlander, G. Lesser, L. Meringoff, T. Robertson, J. Rossiter, and S. Ward. 1977. *Research on the Effects of Television Advertising on Children.* Washington, DC: National Science Foundation.

Barcus, F. Earle. 1975. *Weekend Commercial Children's Television.* Cambridge, MA: Action for Children's Television.

BAR/LNA. 1977. *Ad $ spending.* New York: TNSMI/CMR.

———. 2004. *Ad $ spending.* New York: TNSMI/CMR.

Beales, J. Howard. 1978. An Analysis of Exposure to Non-network Television Advertising. Children's Advertising Rulemaking Comment, Submitted to the Federal Trade Comission.

Biskind, Peter. 1998. Hot Summer Nights. *Newsweek:* A Century on Screen 131(25A): 96–99.

Byrd-Bredbenner, Carol. 2002. Saturday morning children's television advertising: A longitudinal content analysis. *Family and Consumer Sciences Research Journal* 30(3): 382–403.

Cabletelevision Advertising Bureau. 2006a. 2005 cable tv facts, 84% of all television homes receive cable programming. Available at http://www.onetvworld.org/?module=displaystory&story_id=1160&format=html (accessed 16 September 2006).

———. 2006b. 2005 cable tv facts, cable growth charts summary. Available at http://www.onetvworld.org/?module=displaystory&story_id=1154&format=html (access 16 September 2006).

———. 2006c. 2005 cable tv facts, the big erosion picture: Ad-supported cable vs. all broadcast. Available at http://www.onetvworld.org/?module=displaystory&story_id=1257&format=html (accessed 16 September 2006).

———. 2006d. 2005 cable tv facts, the number of ad-supported cable networks with 80%+ tv hh penetration have practically doubled in past year. Available at http://www.onetvworld.org/?module=displaystory&story_id=1158&format=html (accessed 16 September 2006).

———. 2006e. Advertising expenditures, tv market share reports, 4q '04 tv market share for three mediums. Available at http://www.onetvworld.org/?module=displaystory&story_id=1225&format=html (accessed 16 September 2006).

Center for Disease Control and Prevention. National Center for Health Statistics. Prevalence of Overweight Among Children and Adolescents: United States, 20032004. Available: http://www.cdc.gov/nchs/products/pubs/pubd/hestats/obese03_04/ overwght_child_03.htm (accessed 9 June 2006).

Center for Science in the Public Interest. 2003. *Pestering Parents: How Food Companies Market Obesity to Children.* Washington, DC: Center for Science in the Public Interest.

———. 2005. *Guidelines for Responsible Food Marketing Kids.* Washington, DC: Center for Science in the Public Interest. Available: http://www.cspinet.org/marketingguidelines.pdf (accessed 22 September 2006).

Children's Advertising Review Unit. 2006. *Self-regulatory program for children's advertising.* New York: Children's Advertising Review Unit.

Chou, Shin-Yi, Inas Rashad, and Michael Grossman. 2005. Fast-Food Restaurant Advertising on Television and its Influence on Childhood Obesity. NBER Working Paper No. 11879.

FTC/DHHS. 2006. Perspectives on marketing, self-regulation, and childhood obesity. A Report on a Joint Workshop of the Federal Trade Commission and the Department of Health and Human Services, held July 14–15, 2005.

Gantz, Walter, Nancy Schwartz, James Angelini, and Victoria Rideout. 2007. *Food for Thought: Television Food Advertising to Children in the United States.* Menlo Park, CA: Henry J. Kaiser Family Foundation.

Hastings, Gerard, Martine Stead, Laura McDermott, Alasdair Forsyth, Anne Marie MacKintosh, Mike Rayner, Christine Godfrey, Martin Caraher, and Kathryn Angus. 2003. Review of Research on the Effects of Food Promotion to Children. Center for Social Marketing, University of Strathclyde, Glasgow, UK.

Institute of Medicine. 2005. *Preventing Childhood Obesity: Health in the Balance.* Washington, DC: National Academis Press.

Kimmelman, Gene. 2004. Testimony of Gene Kimmelman of Consumers Union before the Committee on Energy and Congress, U.S. House of Representatives, July 14, 2004. Available: http://energycommerce.house.gov/108/Hearings/07142004hearing1336/Kimmelman2 137. htm (accessed 9 November 2006).

Kotz, Krista, and Mary Story. 1994. Food Advertisements During Children's Saturday Morning Television Programming: Are They Consistent with Dietary Recommendations? *Journal of American Dietic Association* 94(11): 12961300.

Kunkel, Dale, and Walter Gantz. 1992. Children's Television Advertising in the Multi-Channel Environment. *Journal of Communication* 42(3):134-152.

Moore, Elizabeth S. 2006. *Its child's play: Advergaming and the online marketing of food to children.* Menlo Park, CA: Henry J. Kaiser Family Foundation.

Ogden, Cynthia L., Margaret D. Carroll, Lester R. Curtin, Margaret A. McDowell, Carolyn J. Tabak, and Katherine M. Flegal. 2006. Prevalence of Overweight and Obesity in the United States, 1999-2004. JAMA 295(13):1549-1555. http://jama.ama-assn.org/cgi/reprint/295/13/1549.pdf.

Ogden, Cynthia L., Katherine M. Flegal, Margaret D. Carroll, and Clifford L. Johnson. 2002. Prevalence and Trends in Overweight Among US Children and Adolescents, 1999-2000. JAMA 288:17281732.

Rideout, Victoria, and Elizabeth Hamel. 2006. *The Media Family: Electronic Media in the Lives of Infants, Toddlers, Preschoolers and their Parents.* Menlo Park, CA: Henry J. Kaiser Family Foundation.

Roberts, Donald, Ulla Foehr, and Victoria Rideout. 2005. *Generation M: Media in the Lives of 8-18 Year-olds.* Menlo Park, CA: Henry J. Kaiser Family Foundation.

Shifrin, Donald. 2005. Remarks during Federal Trade Commission Workshop, "Perspectives on Marketing, Self-Regulation, and Childhood Obesity," July 1415, 2005, Washington, DC. Available: http://www.aap.org/advocacy/washing/dr_%20Shifrin_remarks.htm (accessed 22 September 2006).

Stevenson, Merrill. 1981. The Wiring of Madison Avenue. *The Economist* (U.S. Edition, November 17).

Television Bureau of Advertising. 2006a. Media trends track, tv basics, reach: Broadcast vs. cable. Available at http: //www.tvb. org/rcentral/mediatrendstrack/tvbasics/10_Reach_BdcstvsCable.asp (accessed 23 Nov. 2006).

———. 2006b. Media trends track, tv basics: Time spent viewing - persons. Available at http: //www.tvb. org/rcentral/mediatrendstrack/tvbasics/09_TimeViewingPersons.asp (accessed 16 September 2006).

INDEX

M

N

O

P

Q

R

S

Surgeon General, 47
sweets, 31, 77
symbols, 31
syndicated, 79, 147, 154, 202, 203
systems, 69

T

tangible, 24
targets, 27, 28, 126
task force, 38, 67, 71, 72
taste, 16, 93
tea, 84
teacher training, 13
technology, 37, 55, 59, 60, 69, 92
teenagers, 77, 134, 135, 202
teens, 12, 32, 109, 126, 134, 135, 177, 201
telecommunications, 164
telecommunications services, 164
telephone, 55, 69
television ads, 13, 14, 104, 110, 112, 144
television advertisements, 96, 109, 156, 162
television commercial, 14
television stations, 141
television viewing, 14, 97, 99, 105, 106, 108, 111, 115, 118, 119, 135, 160, 202, 203
test scores, 84
Texas, 78
The Economist, 203, 210
thinking, 35, 57
thresholds, 39
TIA, 69
time periods, 119
tobacco, 75
tofu, 162
toys, 12, 13, 22, 59, 77, 99, 101, 105, 106, 121, 122, 123, 124, 125, 131, 132, 134, 135, 138, 139, 140, 141, 142, 143, 152, 153, 157, 162, 174, 177, 178, 180, 181, 192, 193, 195, 199, 202, 206
tracking, 28, 62, 63
trade, 38, 50, 71
training, 13
trans, 17, 20, 25
transcript, 73

transparency, 65, 70
transparent, 6, 41, 68
travel, 164
trend, 19, 74, 103, 161
triggers, 61
type II diabetes, 9

U

UK, 209
uniform, 12
United States, vii, 1, 8, 9, 64, 73, 84, 91, 208, 209
universities, 69
updating, 5, 37
USDA, 8, 9, 21, 25, 74, 84, 85, 86, 163

V

values, 31
variable, 160
variation, 110, 160, 195
vegetables, 18, 23, 30, 32, 33, 84
video games, 2, 12, 13, 14, 42, 66, 71, 72, 200, 206
viewing patterns, 79, 106, 161
violence, 54
visible, 13, 34, 68, 203
vitamins, 59
vocabulary, 55
voice, 73

W

Wall Street Journal, 82
warrants, 7
watches, 86
water, 17, 26, 83, 84
web, 13, 24, 79
websites, 14, 24, 36, 37, 42, 66, 83, 91, 103, 160
weight loss, 10, 75
weight management, 80

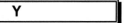

Y